How *to* Look Hot *in a* Minivan

A REAL WOMAN'S GUIDE

to Losing Weight, Looking Great,

and Dressing Chic in the

Age of the Celebrity Mom

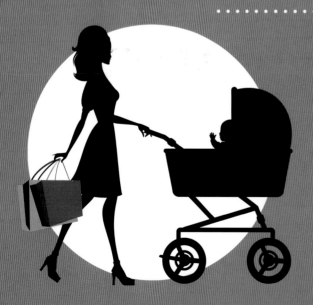

How *to* Look Hot *in a* Minivan

· · · · · ·

JANICE MIN

St. Martin's Press
New York

HOW TO LOOK HOT IN A MINIVAN. Copyright © 2012 by Janice Min. All rights reserved. Printed in China. For information, address St. Martin's Press, 175 Fifth Avenue, New York, N.Y. 10010.

www.stmartins.com

A portion of the text on pages 78, 88–90, and 98–101 has been
repurposed from *Us Hair* 2009. Copyright © 2009 Us Hair LLC.
All Rights Reserved.
Reprinted by Permission.

Design by Susan Walsh

Library of Congress Cataloging-in-Publication Data

Min, Janice.
  How to look hot in a minivan : a real woman's guide to losing weight, looking great, and dressing chic in the age of the celebrity mom / Janice Min. — 1st ed.
      p. cm.
                     ISBN 978-0-312-65897-7 (hbk.)
                     ISBN 978-1-4299-6058-8 (e-book)
   1. Beauty, Personal—Popular works. 2. Mothers—Health and hygiene—Popular works. I. Title.
RA778.M636 2012
646.70085'2--dc23   2011045691

First Edition: September 2012

10 9 8 7 6 5 4 3 2 1

To my husband, Peter, and three kids,
Will, Tate, and Lila,
who always make extra pounds, no sleep,
and bad hair days seem insignificant

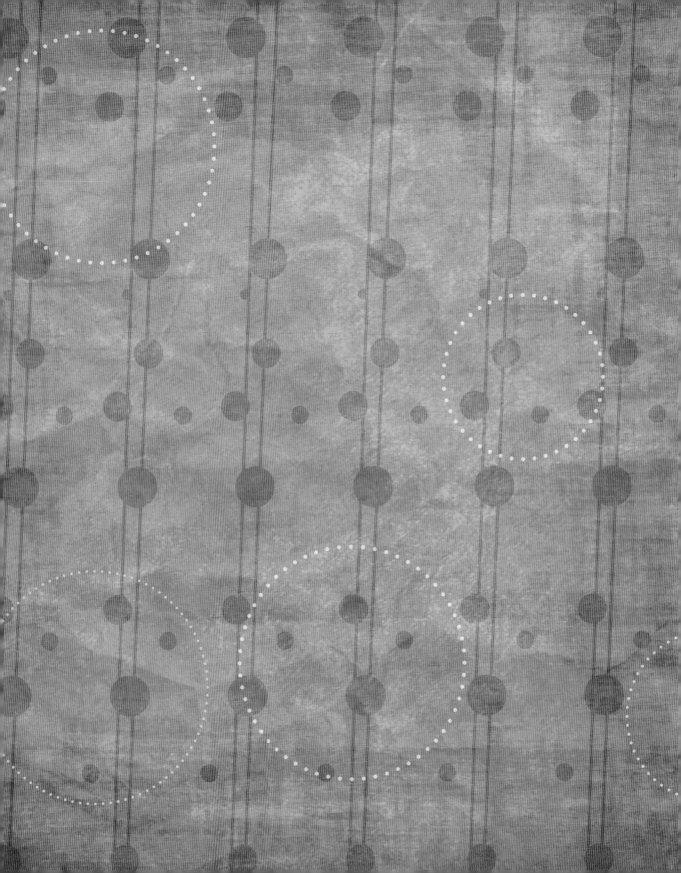

contents

How *to* Look Hot *in a* Minivan

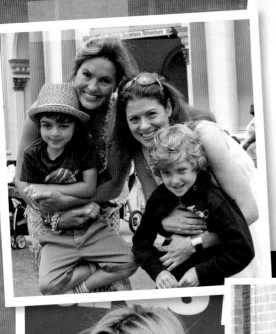

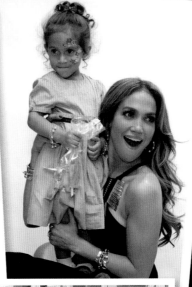

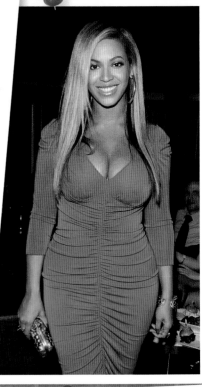

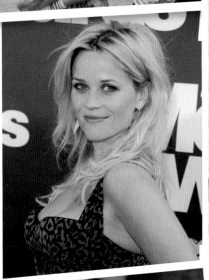

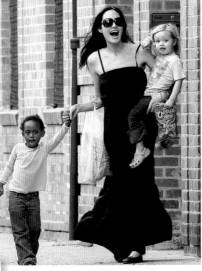

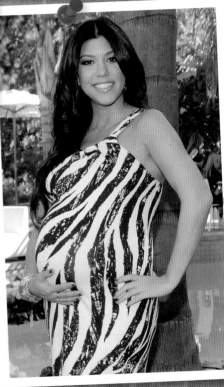

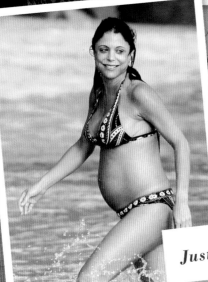

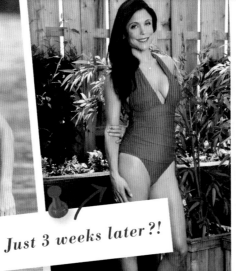

Just 3 weeks later?!

the birth of a trend

It was the summer of 2003. I had just taken over the top job at *Us Weekly* magazine, and my staff and I were noticing the beginnings of a seismic cultural shift: Not only were an unprecedented number of top actresses suddenly pregnant (Courteney Cox, Brooke Shields, Gwyneth Paltrow, Debra Messing, and Denise Richards, to name a few), but they were— for the first time in history—well, *flaunting* it. Whereas less than a decade earlier it had been de rigueur for even the most famous faces to shun the spotlight while expecting (anyone remember how even Madonna, while pregnant with first baby Lourdes, kept herself out of sight?), now practically half of Hollywood was trotting out with a growing tummy and a resplendent pair of golden globes. Seemingly overnight, being "with child" had changed from something synonymous with modesty—even slight embarrassment—to an exciting style statement. Bugaboos became status symbols. Designer cribs went north of $3,000. (We even published photos of a celeb mom favorite, a Lucite crib embedded with *actual* leaves and flowers.) And Pilates and Bikram yoga became pre- and postnatal staples.

The once frumpy bump industry was suddenly big business.

That trend quickly trickled down... to all 82.5 million moms in the country. At school drop-offs, PTA meetings, and suburban Starbucks from coast to coast, American mothers were undergoing a sort of subliminal group makeover. "Mom jeans" were replaced with low-rise, skinny-leg denim; trendy "it" handbags dangled off manicured hands; and one Beverly Hills plastic surgeon even started offering the "Rodeo Drive Mommy Makeover" (a combination tummy tuck and breast augmentation). The idea of a youthful, sexual mother was no longer met with tsk-tsks and disapproval, and—love them or hate them—words like *cougar, yummy mummy,* and *MILF* entered the lexicon. The fashionable mom was in fashion. The age of the "*mom*shell" was born.

Something else, it turns out, was brewing in that fateful, sweltering summer. Just eight weeks after becoming the *Us Weekly* editor-in-chief, I learned that I, too, was pregnant. I was thrilled, of course. I'd put off having children a little longer than the average woman (I was thirty-four) and had no idea what might happen when my husband and I tried to conceive. Those first few months, however, just weren't pretty. I stuffed my formerly fit self into my regular (rapidly shrinking) clothes until finally revealing the news at sixteen weeks. I developed the pimply, problem skin of a sullen adolescent. And to top it all off, I was mortified when the *New York Times* ran a profile of me to document the big promotion. The article, actually, was highly flattering—the picture, however, was not. Pregnant face? I had it. And it wasn't just in my head: A "friend" called to point out just how fat I really looked. (It was a good hazing into the world of maternal insecurities to follow—the worst photo ever taken of me had just run in the most important newspaper in the world. Ugh.)

I started ogling, with morbid fascination, the photographs that flooded my office—red carpet and paparazzi shots of celebrities in bikinis and bandage dresses mere weeks after giving birth. How did these women do it? I wondered. I'd stare at my own ever-expanding body. Then I'd stare at Heidi Klum (who gave birth to a beautiful baby girl one month before my due date and managed to bounce back before I'd even hit the delivery room). I

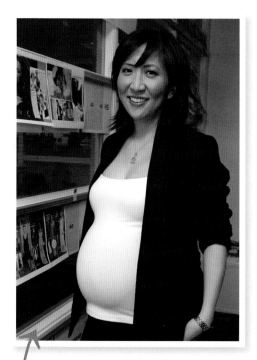

That's me, at Us Weekly, *eight months pregnant with my second son.*

Expecting. Even as an educated woman with access to top style experts and fitness gurus through my line of work, I hadn't fully processed the fact that the female body, after carrying a child around for nine long months, will just never look the same. Obviously, I knew that I'd be gaining some weight, but I just assumed that I'd squeeze it all out in the delivery room, work out a little, and then be back to strolling around SoHo in skinny jeans. A charming, though idiotic, assumption.

think I was in a state of denial; the more I looked at pictures of new celebrity mommies, the more I thought that *this* was just how nature worked. One day you'd look as though you swallowed a basketball. The next day it would be gone. Ta-da!

I don't know about you, but nobody ever told me how difficult it can be to bounce back after baby—not my own mother, not any magazine article, not even that last chapter in *What to Expect When You're*

When I gave birth to my first son, Will, that following spring, I was overcome with joy and gratitude and relief (ten fingers and ten toes? *check*). But after the euphoria of meeting your firstborn fades, there's another big reveal: your postpartum body. The morning after giving birth, I rolled out of bed, dropped my paper-thin hospital robe to the floor, and glanced with some trepidation at myself, stark naked in the mirror. What I saw was something akin to performance art: My stomach had morphed into a deflated, misshapen beach ball. The rest of my body was just sort of oddly toneless, like I'd been molded out of pizza dough. By a preschooler.

With growing terror, I started thinking seriously about that statistic that for every child a woman gives birth to, she puts on something like a permanent ten to fifteen pounds. I recalled the neighborhood moms from my youth in suburban Colorado—women who, with each passing year, grew a little rounder, their bat wings (aka upper-arm flab) a little flappier, the waistbands of their pants a little more elastic. Was I destined to be like that, too? Stuck with the "mom body" I swore I'd never have? I further catastrophized, imagining a day when—years after my kids were grown (or at least out of diapers)—I'd find myself in a Jazzercise class with other middle-aged, out-of-shape ladies, wondering why I was so out of breath. Shudder.

Singer and mom Christina Aguilera once described it like this: "When you have a baby, you go through a period where your body is not your own. It becomes for your child and that's it. It is not for you anymore."

You can say that again. Even after Will's birth, my bladder was still acting like an independent agent, and my breasts had me squirting and spurting in every direction. Yet there was something motivating about the idea of not giving up. Perhaps it's because I had seen firsthand (from a daily barrage of pictures) what was possible after pregnancy; or maybe I was just goosed on by working in the (very

> *You get to the point where you're like, Where am I? What happened to me? I got to get myself together for my kids, you know? They need to know what I really look like!*
>
> —*Jennifer Lopez,*
> *after giving birth to twins Max and Emme*

unforgiving) public eye. Or maybe I was succumbing to a more deep-seated fear: that I had unknowingly stumbled across some unmarked border; that motherhood would change me permanently from "young and fabulous" (though I was never particularly fabulous) to "old and tired." I remember one beautiful summer night in particular—after putting our newborn son to bed, I peered out of our sixth-floor window and saw all these people crowding the streets of New York City's trendy Meatpacking District, just starting to go out to dinner. I panicked. Here I was at home, trapped. My life in all sorts of ways had crossed to the other side.

So maybe my freedom as I'd once known it had come to a screeching halt. But I could still make the most of my nights. Thanks to a cooperative husband, I started running the paths along the West Side Highway, a matrix of public parks in NYC, in the evenings after my son went to sleep. Well, jogging, actually—really, really slowly (again, bladder issues). When Will was six weeks old, I indulged in a personal trainer for the first time in my life. And where I had spent my twenties trying to look "grown-up" by sporting overdone, helmet-head hair and stuffy business suits, now, as a new mom in my mid-thirties, I wanted to look current or *modern* (the word favored

by the well-heeled, trend-obsessed ladies of the magazine's fashion department). I started shopping for clothing with a new, more discerning eye. I was determined to bounce back from pregnancy. I vowed not to let motherhood be an excuse to let myself go.

Sixteen weeks after giving birth, I took a new publicity photo for the magazine (an experience I usually found awkward and uncomfortable). But there was one good thing to come from it. In my favorite outtake from the shoot, I'm wearing a halter-top black dress, sporting one of the best haircuts I've ever had, and in my arms is my newborn son. I remember thinking that I'd pulled something off: Not only did I have a beautiful, healthy baby, but I thought I actually might have looked better than I had *before* I'd gotten pregnant. (Not that I suddenly resembled Heidi Klum, mind you, or any of the other newly minted celebrity mommies; I had accepted that reality a long time ago.) I had become my *own* version of a chic mom—someone polished and put-together, if also a little sleep-deprived. And I profoundly believe that every mother has the (very attainable) dream of radically upping her game, too.

So, okay, I know what you must be thinking. Most moms are too busy, you know, raising children to worry about something so seemingly silly as whether or not their lip gloss is from this season's new line of shades. We rush out the door sans makeup (sometimes still in slippers), comb our daughter's hair before we comb our own (if we comb it at all), and spend what little free time we do have (which amounts to roughly thirty seconds every other Tuesday) daydreaming about how to make a muffin top suddenly disappear. We spend the majority of our disposable income on diapers and day care and baby shoes and burp cloths. And we look at those other, more put-together moms on TV and in magazines—or perhaps even in the car-pool lane—with envy and admiration. Being a mom is hard enough, and now you're telling me that I have to look "cute" while my toddler pelts me with Cheerios from her high chair?

In a word (or two), why not? But the difficulty, I think, isn't that skinny jeans are so hard to get back into; it's that more and more harried mothers feel the need to martyr themselves out of guilt, to put the needs of their children, husband, other moms, and even the family dog ahead of their own. We're *so* concerned with making sure our kids are content, in fact, that we've radically increased the amount of time we spend with them. (A study covered by the *New York Times* reported that mothers today devote around 21.2 hours to child care each week—nearly double what it was in the years before 1995. This, even as more and more women are joining the workforce. And it *still* never feels like enough!) When I just need a break on the weekend, for example, and I let the boys play with their Nintendo Wii, I feel guilty. If a vegetable wasn't cut up to serve with their dinner—even though I grew up on Pringles, bologna, and a diet of partially hydrogenated oils—I feel guilty. If I read them only one book before bed, I feel guilty. And who among us hasn't felt a pang of guilt while sneaking off to get a manicure when we "should" have been with our kids?

The irony, I think, is that in this age of Tiger Mom and *Toddlers & Tiaras*, of logging miles on your minivan carting kids from soccer practice to swim lessons, of dropping hundreds of dollars on ACT training and SAT prep—all in an effort to make our *children* successful—the best thing we can do for our kids might actually be to pay a little more attention to ourselves. Countless studies have concluded that stressed-out, harried moms produce stressed-out, harried kids. Maternal stress has even been linked to weight gain, asthma, and—get this—*shyness* in children.

(Who knew?) And in a landmark study published in 2000, Dr. Ellen Galinsky, president of the Families and Work Institute in New York, asked more than one thousand children about their "one wish" for their parents. Did they ask for more time with mom and dad, as parents perhaps expected (or maybe secretly hoped)? Nope. Instead, "kids were more likely to wish that their parents were less tired and less stressed," Dr. Galinsky said. Remember the Free-Range Kid's movement? What if, just once in a while, you turned yourself into a Free-Range Mom?

This book, though, is not about adding yet another element of stress to your already overpacked life. It's not about resorting to Botox or plastic surgery to look like some ridiculous version of Malibu Mommy Barbie or becoming a cocktail-swilling, Christian Louboutin–wearing, "Real Housewife" of your own town. It's not about denying your role as a mother or putting your children's needs behind your own. And it's not about holding up the "celebrity mom" as some kind of paragon, a woman you should measure yourself against and compare yourself to. (Don't do that. Don't compare yourself to Angelina Jolie. She probably has even Heidi Klum wondering how she does it. And vice versa.)

Rather, this book is about finding ways to reclaim your body and your looks so that you feel your best after birth. And there are plenty of women who could use help with that. According to a recent survey of British moms, for example, a whopping 63 percent said they let themselves go after childbirth, failing to take care of their hair, makeup, and clothes. The majority of women polled also admitted that their confidence took a nosedive when they realized their wardrobe no longer fit. If you're one of the approximately 10 million single or divorced moms in America—and therefore in the throes of dating—the pressure to get your body and looks back could be even greater. Luckily getting back to normal is easier than you might think!

Want to know why some moms seem to bounce back from pregnancy faster than others? I've brought together the top experts in fitness, diet, beauty, and fashion to explain what really happens to your body after baby and reveal the simplest (and most cost-effective) ways to become a thinner, better-looking, and even sexier mom. Together, we'll uncover the secrets behind the stars' seemingly effortless style, and I'll also debunk some post-pregnancy myths (because any woman who said she lost the baby weight just by "running around after her kids" is *lying to you*).

I'll let you in on a little secret: I never aspired to work at a celebrity magazine or ever much cared about celebrities—in fact, as a somewhat nerdy teenager who always won the current events quiz, I imagined one day becoming a White House correspondent. And I've never been much of a girly-girl. I wasn't raised with the idea that women are "supposed" to get regular mani-pedis, or pay someone to pluck their brows, or not have hairy arms. I didn't get my first manicure until I was well into my twenties, which is right around the time I finally learned how to distinguish Max Azria from T.J. Maxx. (Left to my own devices, without the pressure of social convention, I imagine I would easily slide into sweats and a ponytail 24/7.) In a twist of fate, however, it was running a celebrity magazine that taught me that looking great isn't just for the rich, the pampered, or the lucky. Being a "hot mom"—or even just a presentable one—is really about achieving one's potential. We ask that of our kids and our husbands, right? We should feel good about asking that of ourselves.

With just a little help, you *can* get back to being the woman you were pre-pregnancy—even if you're driving a minivan!

who looked even better after baby

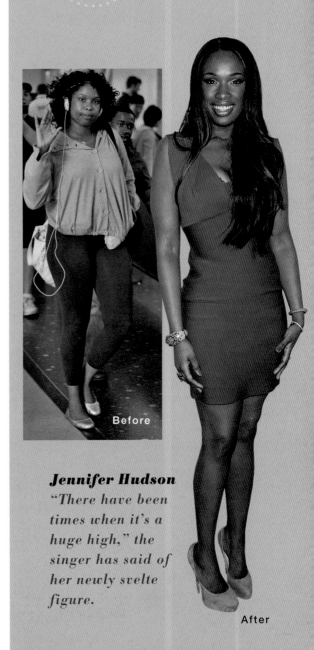

Before

Jennifer Hudson
"There have been times when it's a huge high," the *singer has said of her newly svelte figure.*

After

These hot celebrity mamas came back looking more fit and stylish *after giving birth.*

Gwen Stefani

The chic rocker/ designer says of her two boys, "Being a mom was all I ever dreamed about."

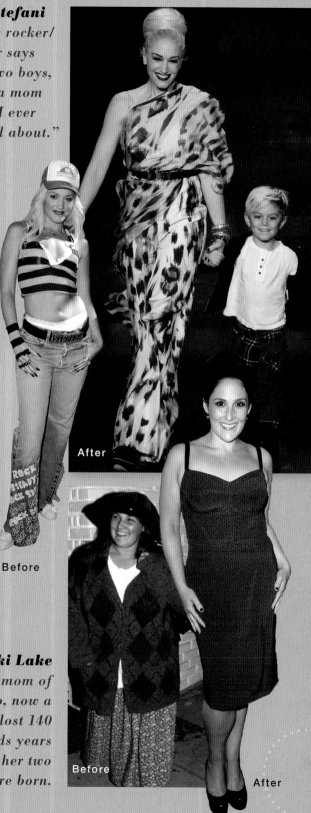

After

Before

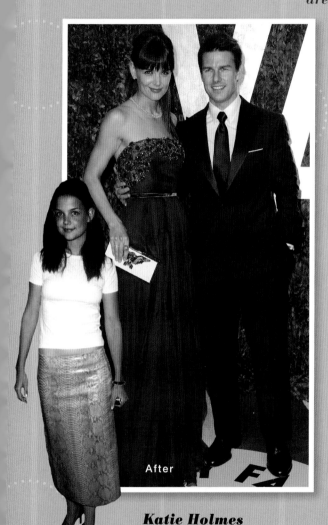

After

Before

Katie Holmes

The actress has said she buys clothes thinking one day her daughter might wear them.

Ricki Lake

The mom of two, now a size 6, lost 140 pounds years after her two sons were born.

Before

After

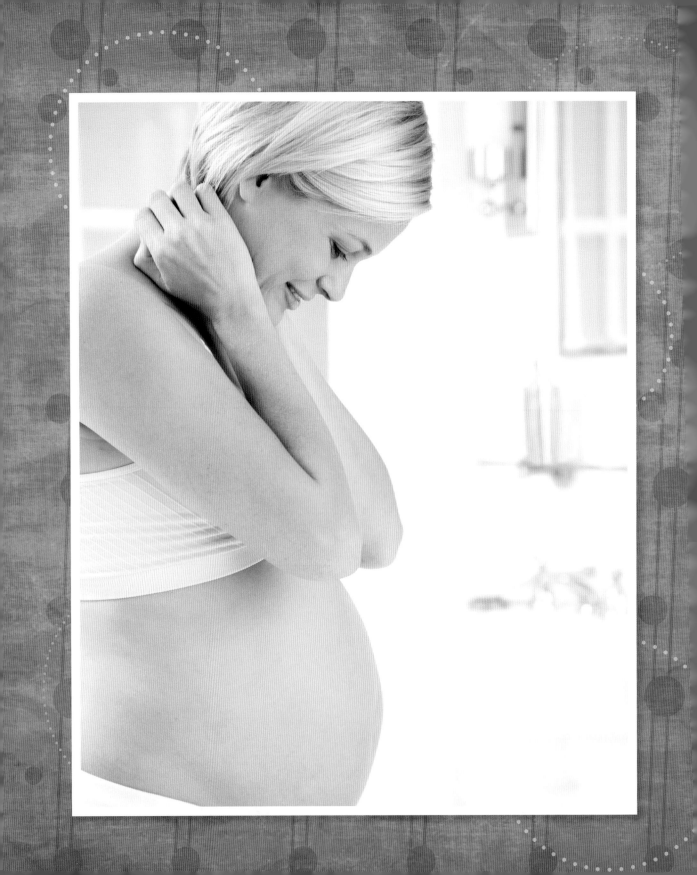

what i didn't expect after expecting

The 10 Terrible Things That Happen Postpartum

The morning after I gave birth to my first son, Will (the same morning I realized my stomach had morphed into something resembling a pool toy), I gathered the courage to step on the scale. Happily, I discovered that I'd already lost twenty-five of the thirty pounds I'd put on during pregnancy. Victory! Within weeks, I was still flabby, but I was back in my regular clothes (and, admittedly, feeling a little superior about that). Twenty-three months later, I delivered a second son, Tate—in the same hospital, no less—and I smugly hopped on the scale expecting the same results. I think I just assumed that I was one of those "lucky" women with good genes who would bounce back to my normal weight with little to no work. Unfortunately, I was not. I'd just had a six-pound, ten-ounce baby boy, but I was only *seven* pounds lighter than I'd been before giving birth.

I actually stepped off and back on the scale at least four times, just to make sure it wasn't broken. It wasn't. I still had twenty-three pounds to go, and seemingly all of them were centered in the middle of my gut (every new mom knows the feeling; it's the perma-five-months-pregnant look). Losing the baby weight would prove much more difficult the second time around.

In fact, I was riding the New York City subway to work one morning, right around the time I came back from maternity leave, when an older gentleman repeatedly offered me his seat. I realized in horror that he thought I was *still* pregnant. And even though he was trying to be kind, the attempt at

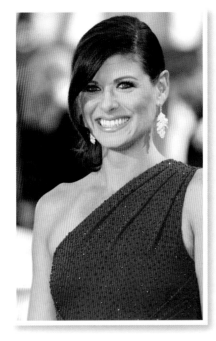

One year after I gave birth, I hadn't lost all my baby weight. People were like, She's pregnant. And I was like, Nope—I'm just fat! I'm not one of those girls who can lose all that weight in six weeks, and, by the way, who are those people?

—Actress and mom Debra Messing

chivalry made me sort of hate him—not to mention feel absolutely ashamed of the way I looked. Not long after that, I was vacationing with my family when some bizarre woman approached me, told me she was "psychic," stared at my stomach, and asked if I was pregnant. (I wasn't.) After *that,* I was with my kids at a petting zoo when someone else asked me how far along I was. For seven long months, people would periodically ask if I was expecting and completely ruin my day in the process. (This is why I will never, *ever* ask a woman if she's pregnant—unless she's actually being wheeled into a maternity ward.)

I remember waiting for some kind of miracle to happen, for my old metabolism to "kick in" or my hormones to straighten out—anything that would help rid me of that postnatal paunch. Despite the old adage that breastfeeding will help the pounds "melt away," the baby weight just wouldn't budge (and I nursed for fourteen whole months!). I even had my thyroid tested, more than half hoping I had some kind of legitimate health problem. It was enough to make me want to hide at home (not an option, unfortunately) or just give up altogether. I felt like I was teetering on the precipice of just letting it all go. Why even try when nothing seemed to work?

> **Sometimes I look at old pictures of myself and I think, Aaagh! I need to get that back.**
>
> **—Reality star and mom Kendra Wilkinson** *on life after childbirth*

Thankfully, I discovered that I wasn't alone—lots of women *think* they're prepared for the aftermath of pregnancy, but most are in for a really rude awakening. That abracadabra I'm-back-in-a-bikini tap dance that celebrities do, usually between three and six *weeks* postpartum, is just not in the cards for the average woman (and, of course, it completely distorts our expectations for ourselves).

"I think we're all a bit sheltered from the realities of life after childbirth," says New York OB-GYN Shari Brasner, M.D. "For example, if a woman has an abdomen that's incredibly scarred by stretch marks, she probably isn't showing it off in a bikini at the beach." New York dermatologist David Colbert, who counts celebrity moms Angelina Jolie and Naomi Watts as clients, agrees: "I've often said that we should have pre-pregnancy support groups, where we explain to women: *This* is what will happen to your body. Women need to be informed and prepared, because if you're not, it's like bungee jumping."

Well, I know I certainly bungee jumped into motherhood—and if you felt like crying because Skinnygirl Bethenny Frankel somehow managed to don her size 4 bathing suit just *twenty-one days* after giving birth, you probably bungee jumped, too. And let's be realistic: Somewhere along the way we all got tricked into thinking that no matter what we looked like before baby, we would bounce back looking like smoking-hot Jessica Alba. Not gonna happen. Most women are not rubber bands that just snap back in place after having a baby. In fact, your body—no matter how hard you work out or how many pounds you shed— will probably always look a little different after you give birth. Not worse, necessarily, but different. And it's important to understand all the ways your body likely has changed *before* you attempt to get back in your skinny jeans (and beat yourself up if you can't). Right off the bat, I thought it would be helpful to explain exactly what we're dealing with. So here's what can you expect…after you've finished expecting.

Rapid and Sudden Hair Loss

Remember how gloriously thick your hair felt during pregnancy? Then, just a few months after giving birth—*wham!*—you're suddenly shedding like a sheepdog. It's not uncommon for new moms to develop a little halo of "baby hairs" around the forehead and the hairline or to feel as though they're losing more hair than normal. For months after I gave birth, I would torture myself in the shower, counting just how many hairs had fallen out into my hands, calculating how long I had left before the inevitable baldness set in. And I wasn't the only one who noticed: Once, I was getting made up for a TV appearance, when the makeup artist announced that he was going to dust dark brown eye shadow onto the part in my hair so that it would look "less wide." Horrifying.

So what's the deal with this sudden succession of bad hair days? Everybody sheds a little bit; in fact, typical hair loss is about one hundred strands per day. During pregnancy, however, elevated levels of estrogen in your body prolong the growth phase of the individual hairs, making them grow longer before they fall out. When your hormones eventually return to their pre-pregnancy levels, usually somewhere around four to six months postpartum, the normal hair loss cycle returns, too, in a process medically referred to as "telogen effluvium." "All those hairs that synchronized in the growth part of the cycle are now entering the loss phase together," says Dr. Brasner. That's when you'll start to feel as though you're suddenly going bald.

Though in most cases post-pregnancy hair loss will resolve on its own, it can sometimes be exacerbated by a thyroid condition, such as postpartum thyroiditis or severe postpartum iron-deficiency anemia (tests for both can be performed at your OB-GYN's office). In the meantime, you can help keep your hair healthy by using a conditioner and a detangler, rather than yanking at stubborn knots, and by not pulling your hair up in a high, tight ponytail (which can cause added strain at the hairline as well as additional breakage). "Since some of my patients want to be proactive while waiting for their hair growth to kick in," adds Dr. Brasner, "I sometimes prescribe iron supplements, even if their iron levels are relatively normal." If you feel that you're suffering from excessive hair loss, don't hesitate to speak with your doctor.

"Momnesia"

I used to have a near photographic memory. I could recite phone numbers without ever having to look them up, knew all my credit card numbers by heart, and had such detailed recall of events and conversations that more than one of my friends described my ability as "elephantine." Now, I seriously can't remember a thing. I create passwords for all my online accounts and mere moments later have no idea what I typed. Sometimes when I'm traveling for work, I actually have to stop and think about which airport I'm in. I even managed to leave my purse in the American Airlines lounge in New York once…and didn't realize it until I had landed in California.

If having a baby has made you a little scatterbrained, you're not alone. Recent research suggests that "maternal amnesia"—with symptoms including, most commonly, an increase in forgetfulness, clumsiness, anxiety, stress, or the inability to concentrate—is a legitimate phenomenon among new mothers. (Though the prevalence of buzzing, vibrating devices and nonstop Internet access doesn't help. These days it's almost impossible to focus on one thing at a time. And it drives me crazy that any device that makes a beep or buzz—BlackBerrys, iPhones, etc.—somehow *must*

be acknowledged by its owner, even in the middle of a conversation. Horrible.)

But don't let the term *amnesia* scare you—it's not as though you suddenly won't be able to recognize your own husband. However, according to a study published in the *Journal of Clinical and Experimental Neuropsychology,* performing *new* memory tasks, like learning a new phone number or remembering a new acquaintance's name (or recalling where in the world you put the pacifier that your baby wants *right this minute*), may prove slightly more difficult than before you got pregnant.

Researchers aren't sure what causes "mom brain," but it's thought that a variety of factors, including sleep deprivation, hormonal fluctuations, and the general upheaval that occurs when you bring baby home from the hospital, probably contribute to this phenomenon of forgetfulness. Also, symptoms may be present for up to one year after giving birth (though I think it probably lasts well beyond that), so while you're busy adjusting to your new role as a mom, you may want to actually start *using* the calendar on your iPhone or plastering your walls with Post-its. And try not to be too hard on yourself when and if you forget things. It happens.

The Mask of Pregnancy

It's not uncommon for pregnant women to develop a condition called "melasma," a form of hyperpigmentation (or discoloration of the skin) that most often appears on the upper lip, cheeks, and forehead. In fact, the American Academy of Dermatology reports that up to 70 percent of pregnant women will develop "the mask of pregnancy," as it's more commonly known. (And that 70 percent includes me—I had what looked like an ink spill on my forehead, as well as a darker patch on my upper lip that *still* shows up in just the slightest bit of sun. Unfortunately, it closely resembles Hitler's trademark mustache.)

Melasma is caused by a combination of sun exposure

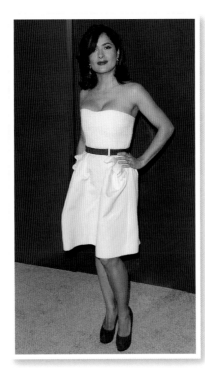

I thought, I'm just going to lose all the weight superfast because I'm going to breastfeed, and everybody tells you that if you breastfeed, it's going to come off like this. It's a lie!

—Actress and mom Salma Hayek

and an increase in the hormones estrogen and progesterone (which means that it can also show up on women who are taking birth control pills, since the oral contraceptive triggers an increase in those same hormones). While makeup tends to make the discoloration look worse (my husband once asked me with alarm, "What is *on your face?*" after I tried to cover it with foundation), it is possible for the spots to fade on their own after childbirth or when you stop taking the pill. Older, more stubborn patches may require a topical treatment, like a skin-lightening or retinoid cream or laser treatments (more on that in chapter 7). Meanwhile, protect your skin with a sunblock (not just sunscreen) containing zinc or titanium dioxide.

Shrunken, Droopy, and Misshapen Breasts

If you think your breasts are smaller now than they were pre-pregnancy, they probably are. Many women experience a decrease in cup size around the time they finish breastfeeding. "I call this the 'shrivel up and disappear' phenomenon," says Dr. Brasner. "It's most common in women who are very thin, because they had very little fat in their breasts to begin with. But it's impossible to predict who will experience 'shrinkage.'"

So what causes this dreaded deflation? When progesterone and estrogen levels rise during pregnancy, all the inner structures of the breast glands increase, including the alveoli (where the milk is made and stored) and the ducts (the route the milk takes before passing out of the nipple). After delivery, however, that tissue starts to undergo some post-pregnancy "remodeling." In about 30 percent of cases, women will eventually see their breasts return to normal size. For the other 70 percent, oral contraceptives may prove helpful, since synthetic hormones often cause "the girls" to grow. Dr. Brasner also points out that your breasts will continue to grow and change with each subsequent pregnancy, so if you're not yet finished having children, there's still a chance that your bustline will bounce back all on its own. And if that doesn't work, well, you can always spring for a well-padded bra.

Speaking of bras, wearing a good one can actually *reduce* the likelihood that your boobs will one day relocate from your chest to your knees. "When your breasts enlarge during pregnancy and breastfeeding, that extra weight creates tension on and damage to the ligaments that support the breasts off the chest wall," says Dr. Brasner. That added strain *could* cause an irreversible sagging, not to mention unsightly stretch marks. "By wearing a supportive bra," Dr. Brasner explains, "you'll reduce the likelihood of permanently stretching out those ligaments." In other words, resist the urge to go all *National Geographic*, even when you're home alone with a nursing newborn.

> *I thought after you had the baby your tummy would just go down. I remember going, What's this deflated, wobbly thing?*
>
> —Actress and mom Rachel Griffiths

Longer, Wider, and Weirder Nipples

It's no secret that breastfeeding will affect the size, shape, and appearance of the nipples (and any woman who has watched in horror as her nipple was stretched out to four inches when inserted in a breast pump probably assumed—correctly, as it turns out—that this outcome was inevitable). "The length of time dedicated to nursing can influence the changes, but most women will notice that their nipples have become wider, or more prominent, or both," says Dr. Brasner. Short of surgery, these changes are permanent.

Stretch Marks

"If you're going to stretch the skin of your abdomen for nine long months," warns dermatologist Dr. Colbert, "*something* is going to happen. Stretch marks are simply a rite of passage." That may be true, but stretch marks—which may appear anywhere you gain weight, in particular on your breasts, hips, thighs, butt, and, of course, stomach—are a major bummer.

Who gets stretch marks is determined largely by genetics, though studies estimate that anywhere from 50 to 90 percent of pregnant woman will develop these unsightly pink scars. "Supermodel Christy Turlington might never get a stretch mark in her whole life," explains Dr. Colbert, "while someone else might develop them just by having her skin gently tugged on. Most of us are somewhere in between." The good news is that stretch marks are somewhat treatable and will improve over time (we'll talk more about that in chapter 4).

Belly Bulge and Muffin Top

The recommended weight gain during pregnancy is around thirty pounds, and roughly eight pounds of that will be fat, most of which is deposited—perhaps not surprisingly—right in the middle of your gut. "It's the hardest fat to lose," says Dr. Brasner. "Most new mothers will feel as though they've thickened around the waist."

Compounding matters is a little-known—but almost universal—muscular injury that occurs during pregnancy. "Diastasis recti" is a separation of the two vertical bands of abdominal muscles that meet in your middle; normally, these muscles help to hold you in, but when they split, you wind up with that protruding "potbelly" look. In more extreme cases (typically after a multiples birth), diastasis recti can even cause your stomach pooch to resemble…well, a derriere. Reality TV star Kate Gosselin, after delivering sextuplets, famously displayed her "butt in the front" on the hit show *Jon and Kate Plus 8* and later underwent a tummy tuck to correct it.

"Almost 100 percent of pregnant women will get diastasis recti," says Dr. Brasner. "Unfortunately, there is little that can be done to prevent it." However, there are a number of exercises that may help you *correct* it. We'll go over those in greater detail in chapter 6.

Some women also will notice a little (or maybe large) pooch of fat in their lower abs, which has nothing to do with diastasis recti or even a swollen uterus (the uterus shrinks to its pre-pregnancy size within six weeks of delivery); if you can pinch more than an inch or so of skin on your lower abdomen, it's fat, plain and simple.

To fight that dreaded muffin top effect (that spillage of fat over the waistband of your pants), you're going to want to pack away your low-rise jeans, at least temporarily. Opt instead for a midrise pair, and don't be afraid to go up a size or two. "If you try to squeeze into too-tight jeans, the muffin top and back fat are only going to make you feel worse about yourself," says Sara Blakely, owner and creator of Spanx shapewear and mom to a toddler. "I went up two sizes in jeans after having my baby, and I'm just now getting back to my pre-pregnancy size."

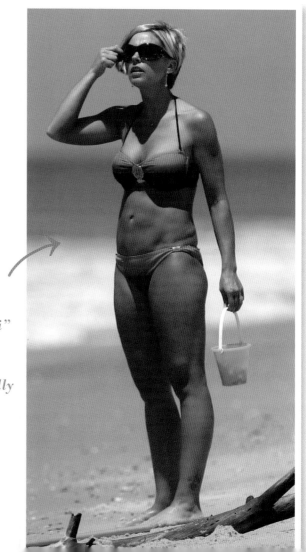

Mom of eight Kate Gosselin, after a tummy tuck to correct "diastasis recti" and sagging skin on her postpartum belly

Enlarged Vagina

Icky, but true: Almost all women who deliver vaginally will notice that their lady bits feel a little, ahem, *stretched out* after childbirth—even if there was no tearing or even after an episiotomy has completely healed. "The tissues of the vagina undergo a fair amount of trauma during delivery," warns Dr. Brasner, and in some cases, those changes may even affect sexual satisfaction when you resume having intercourse.

While some women may be tempted to resort to plastic surgery—in the last five years or so, "vaginal rejuvenation" has seemed to increase exponentially in popularity (at least anecdotally)—many doctors are strongly opposed to these types of controversial procedures. "Many surgical sites claim these operations will enhance your sex life," says Dr. Brasner, "but a healthy woman should be able to accept that these changes are normal and natural. I think doctors who offer these types of procedures are preying on women with low self-esteem."

A better (and certainly cheaper) option? Kegel exercises, which can help tone and tighten the muscles of the pelvic floor. To perform a Kegel, tighten and release the pelvic muscles—the same muscles that you would use to stop the flow of urine—and work up to doing three sets of ten per day. Keep in mind, however, that Kegels will not alter any *exterior* changes, which may include a larger vaginal opening and labia.

I read about these actresses who get on a stationary bike two weeks after giving birth and I'm like, What? Where did you push your baby out? Since having [daughter] Aviana, I have a muffin top, and that's okay.

—Actress and mom Amy Adams

the pee-pee problem

No, I am not talking about your child's issues, but rather your own. "Almost every woman who carries a term pregnancy, regardless of mode of delivery, will describe some change in bladder function after delivery," says Dr. Brasner. "I see this in my office all the time. It could be a change in urge, incontinence with cough or sneeze, or incontinence during activities." Sound familiar? I for one remember doing jumping jacks during a fitness class at the gym shortly after giving birth...and then realizing that probably wasn't a great idea. All of these changes in bladder function are, of course, caused by a weakening of the pelvic floor supports, including soft tissues and ligaments, as a result of childbirth.

Dr. Brasner explains that full bladder function may not return while you're nursing (the tissues of the pelvic floor are very estrogen-dependent, but estrogen levels in your body remain suppressed when you're breastfeeding). Kegel exercises, however, can help some women regain some muscle strength and reduce symptoms. If problems persist, Dr. Brasner points out that there is a growing field of experts in urogynecology, where surgeons specialize in techniques to restore normal anatomy and function to the pelvic floor. And don't hesitate to ask your doctor about medication and alternative treatments (including biofeedback in some cases) that also may help improve incontinence.

Spider Veins

For some unlucky ladies, pregnancy may trigger a sudden outbreak of unsightly, visible veins (of all shapes and sizes) in the legs, the thighs, and even the pubic area. "Spider veins" (small veins, close to the skin's surface, that resemble spiderwebs or tree branches) as well as varicose veins, which are typically large, bulging, and ropy in appearance, are caused by changes in blood circulation that you may experience while expecting.

During pregnancy, the veins in your body begin to enlarge to accommodate an increase in blood flow. Additionally, the weight of your growing baby puts a decent amount of pressure on the vena cava vein—a major blood vessel that runs down the right side of your body. In fact, pregnant women—as you may know—are often encouraged to start sleeping on their left side (typically somewhere around sixteen weeks) to improve circulation as well as relieve the weight of the uterus on the vena cava; this may prove helpful if you're still struggling with varicose veins even after delivery.

Another common variation of vein swelling includes hemorrhoids, which are essentially varicose veins of the rectum. Thankfully, hemorrhoids brought on by

pregnancy tend to disappear quickly. As for visible veins in the legs, about 50 percent of cases will subside once the baby is born, according to Dr. Colbert. To help the process along, try elevating your feet and ankles whenever possible and avoid sitting or standing for long periods of time.

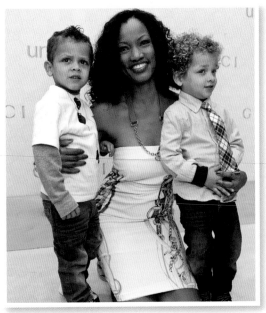

I don't have a six-pack, but if I did, it'd mean I wasn't spending enough time with my kids. So I'm fine with it.

—Actress and mom of three Garcelle Beauvais-Nilon

Spreading Hips, Ribs, and Widening Feet

Even if you've lost the baby weight, you may notice that your clothes just don't fit like they used to. That's because many different body parts expand during pregnancy, and—*sigh*—sometimes they stay that way.

The culprit is the (appropriately named) hormone relaxin, which helps loosen or "relax" the ligaments so that your body can make room for baby. The most obvious place where expansion occurs is, of course, in the pelvic region—the bones slowly spread to make way for a growing fetus, as well as for his or her eventual delivery. (A new study actually shows that—whether you've had kids or not—your hips will continue to widen into your seventies, even as your other bones shrink. Hooray.) Additionally, the baby (and your uterus) occupies a lot of real estate right underneath the rib cage. Organs often get shoved northward, and as anyone who has ever been kicked in the ribs during pregnancy knows, it's a tight squeeze in there. Jennifer Lopez admitted that even though she got back down to her pre-pregnancy dress size, her rib cage was noticeably altered after having twins: "Before, I was always able to fit into sample-size clothes from designers, and now they have to let them out just a bit." (I've had my own issues with clothing; my breasts shrank, yet my ribs expanded, and nothing zips up like it used to. Bummer.)

Just like the hips and ribs, your feet may undergo some major changes during and after pregnancy. The twenty-six bones in each foot have to support a lot of extra weight, and they will often spread out in both width and length, thanks again to relaxin. In fact, doctors estimate that about half of all women will exit pregnancy with permanently larger feet than before. (Oddly, mine ended up a half size smaller, which no doctor ever seems to believe when I've mentioned it.) Anyway, it's a good idea to save any major shoe shopping until at least a month after delivery—give yourself some time to see where things settle.

I returned to work 25 pounds heavier than people are used to seeing me. There was nothing I could do about it. I just thought, I had a baby, that's way more important.

—Top Chef host and mom Padma Lakshmi

why some moms bounce back faster than others

Research shows that the average postpartum weight retention is anywhere from one to six and a half pounds, though some studies put that number as high as ten to fifteen pounds. That means that if you have two children, you could easily wind up twenty pounds heavier than you were on your wedding day. And if you gain more than the recommended twenty-five to thirty pounds during pregnancy (and 36 percent of women do), that number could be even higher. However, the *greatest* indicator of your ability to shed the baby weight isn't how much you gained, it's the shape you were in before you got pregnant. So if you didn't look like Gisele Bündchen before you had kids, it's probably a safe bet that you aren't going to look like her afterward.

"I think that genetics as well as pre-pregnancy levels of fitness play the biggest roles in how quickly women bounce back," says Dr. Brasner. "In my experience, age isn't much of a factor." In other words, a woman who eats a sensible diet and is fit *before* getting pregnant is probably more likely to eat a sensible diet and be fit after delivery. How your own mother coped with her postpartum body also might be an indication of what you can expect in the future. "If a woman's mother was able to return to her pre-pregnancy weight and shape after each delivery," continues Dr. Brasner, "I find that ups the chances that my patient will do the same."

To increase the likelihood that you'll make it back into your skinny jeans, Dr. Brasner recommends trying to lose the baby weight within six months of delivery—especially if you're planning to have more children in the future. A woman who starts a second pregnancy at the same weight as her *first* pregnancy can typically expect to be able to drop the pounds again, while women who don't shed the weight between pregnancies will face a much bigger hurdle. "It really doesn't matter what the interval between pregnancies is," says Dr. Brasner, "it's the *cumulative* weight gains that really add up."

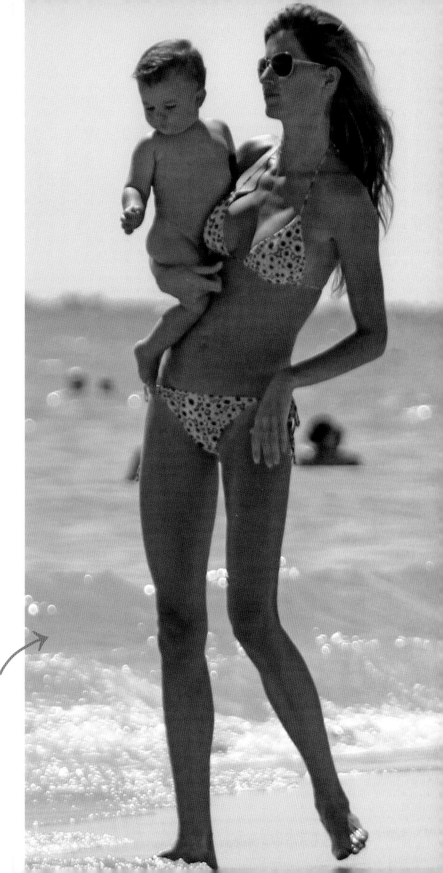

> *I can't ever get down to the weight I was before I had [first child] Honor. My body's just different. The jeans sort of zip up differently, and things hang differently. It's a miracle what happens, but you definitely are different afterward....Unless you're Gisele.*
>
> *—Mom of two Jessica Alba*

Gisele Bündchen hit the beach ten months after giving birth.

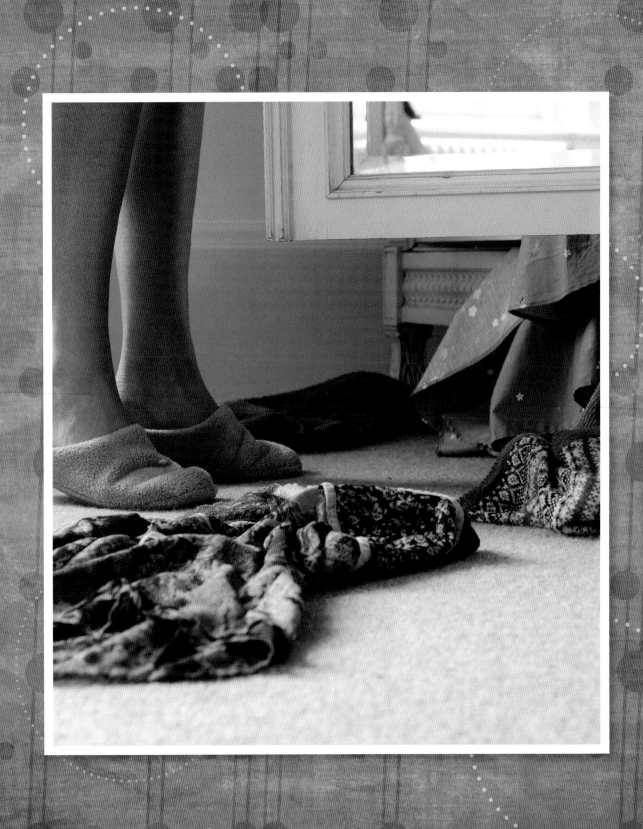

chic and cool for carpool

Style Help for the Harried with Children

Many, many years ago—long before I had kids of my own—I took a job working alongside a frenetic, frantic, and often frazzled mother of two. Every morning she would rush into the office with fresh food stains on her shirt, a shock of hair in various states of frizz, and paperwork spilling out of whatever random shopping bag she happened to be carrying (a plastic grocery sack frequently doubled as some sort of briefcase). She was usually juggling a take-out coffee and economy-size muffin, too, which she would proceed to eat at her desk while spitting out crumbs as she spoke (usually about how brilliant her children were). One morning in particular, however, she regaled me with a story that has haunted me for years: While dropping her child off at school just an hour earlier, she confessed, another mother said something that had left her utterly shocked (though, unfortunately, not speechless). "Please step away from me," this woman at drop-off had said. "Your breath is terrible." And then my colleague launched into a long, drawn-out defense about how she didn't have *time* to brush her teeth in the morning. Why didn't this other busy working mother understand?!

Children or no children, I made a mental note to never let myself become anything like this woman.

If my crazy colleague represented one end of what you might call the "extreme mom spectrum," the mother I encountered a few years later, on the morning I took one of my sons to his first day of school, certainly represented the other—she was an impossibly svelte woman dressed in four-inch stilettos and a tight designer dress (probably a Lanvin), toting an Hermès Birkin bag (they start at around $5,000!), and sporting hair and makeup that was just a little too *done*. All this for an informal playground meeting and a quick talk with the teachers? For the next few days— actually it was weeks—she was referred to simply as "overdressed mom" by other women who'd seen the spectacle. (Even my husband, who is pretty oblivious to mama drama, took notice.)

It's no secret that mothers are under an unprecedented amount of pressure to look young and fresh and fabulous (while making it all look so easy).

In fact, I was on the phone with someone I know recently, a woman with two grown children who lives in a posh New York City suburb, and she reminded me that in "her day," it was perfectly acceptable to schlep around in sweats. ("You should *see* some of the moms these days," she told me of her Prada- and Gucci-clad neighbors.) But what I've discovered over the last few years is this: The mounting expectation on all mothers to up their game seems to have triggered two distinctly different trends. There are those who go overboard, frantically fighting time by pumping their faces full of Botox and dropping thousands on designer fashions and expensive handbags, and then there are some mothers who simply just give up. Perhaps they'll work on self-improvement when the kids are older, they sometimes say. It's like we're living in some kind of warped Freudian fantasy, an updated version of the Madonna/whore complex.

What we're all in need of is a little balance. Surely a look that's polished and put-together can also be easy to pull off without screaming to the world, "I'm trying so hard!" The secret here isn't owning more and stuffing your closet like a Real Housewife of Beverly Hills, but owning the right few pieces—classic, timeless items that will never go out of style. These days more and more retailers are tapping fashion's biggest names (think Missoni for Target, Lanvin's Alber Elbaz designing for H&M, or Vera Wang at Kohl's), making it easier than ever to find well-designed, classic clothes that don't cost a fortune. Even First Lady Michelle Obama recently wowed in a $35 H&M dress that she wore for an appearance on the *Today* show!

I've rounded up some of the top experts to explain the basics of building a wardrobe that can take you from morning carpool to evening cocktails, or conservative boardroom to neighborhood playground. Being a mom doesn't have to suck the life out of your personal style. Let's work on getting your pre-pregnancy groove back.

Your diaper bag doesn't have to be ugly! Turn to page 56 to see what celebrity moms tote around.

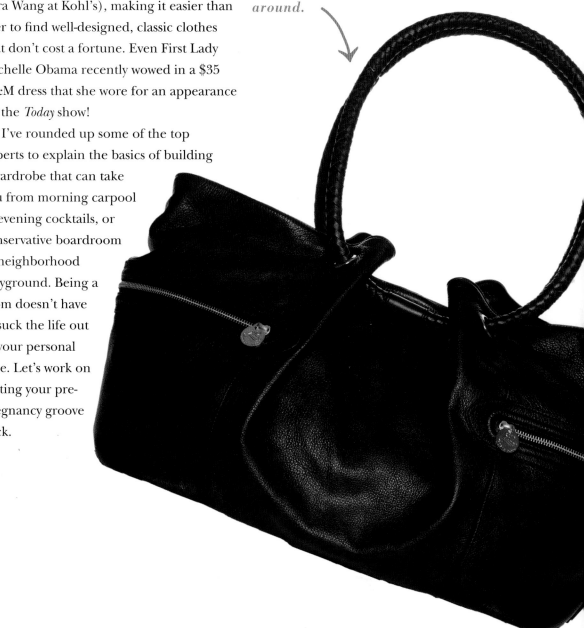

THE top 10 MOM MISHAPS

In 2010, a principal at an elementary school got so fed up with moms wearing pajamas to drop off their kids (as many as 50 a day!) that he sent a scathing letter home with each and every student, calling the practice "slovenly and rude." This, after a grocery store in Wales marched a 24-year-old mother of two out the door for shopping in her PJs and then banned nightwear and slippers from the premises altogether. While that may sound a bit extreme, think how you'd feel if you went to the bank, or your dentist's office, or a law firm, and your teller/doctor/attorney came out to greet you in fuzzy slippers and a bathrobe. You certainly wouldn't send your child to school in pajamas, so why would you allow yourself to laze about in stretchy sweats (all the time, that is)? Below are some common fashion faux pas to avoid. (Disclaimer: I'll admit it. I have been guilty of some of these wardrobe crimes myself. But I try not to make it a habit.)

3 Too Tight After Baby

You're not fooling anyone if the size says "8" but your body says "14." Don't try to squeeze into your pre-pregnancy wardrobe until you're truly ready—you'll only look bigger.

4 Pajamas or Workout Wear

No matter how busy you are, you still have enough time to get dressed in the morning. Find another go-to casual ensemble other than sweats.

2 Crocs

Crocs should not be considered acceptable footwear. A ballet flat is just as comfortable and more fashion-forward.

1 Dressing Like Your Daughter

Even if you and your teenager can wear the same clothes, don't. Sharing clothes with a minor is a definite don't.

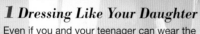

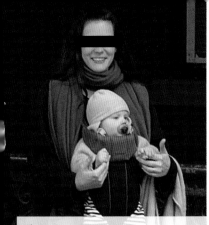

5 Matronly Skirts
Skirts should hit just above or just below the knee—any longer than that and you'll look vaguely Amish.

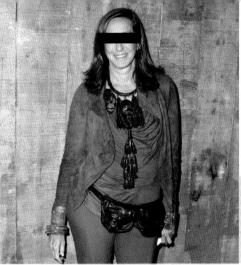

6 Backpack or Fanny Pack as Purse
It doesn't matter how many top designers try to make the fanny pack "cool," it's just not gonna happen. Try a messenger bag if you want to go hands-free.

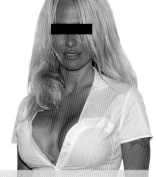
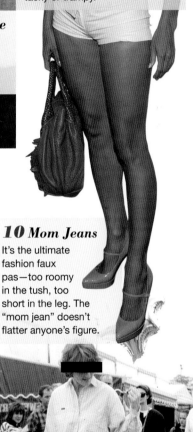

7 The Cougar
Personally, I hate the word *cougar*; it smacks of creepy sexism. But there's just no excuse for dressing tacky or trampy.

9 Exposed Undergarments
Please do not leave the house if you have butt cleavage. And no one wants to see your bra, either. There is nothing sexy about it.

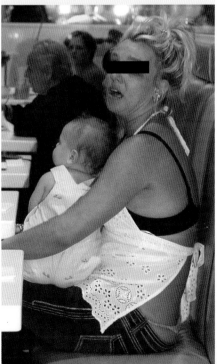

10 Mom Jeans
It's the ultimate fashion faux pas—too roomy in the tush, too short in the leg. The "mom jean" doesn't flatter anyone's figure.

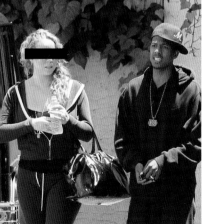

8 Matching Track Suits (and Anything Velour)
It's *so* 1995. Plus, no woman should ever wear something with a designer's logo printed across the bum.

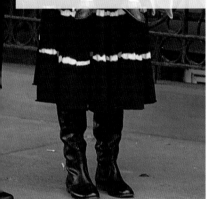

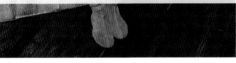

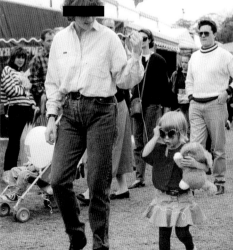

The Best-Dressed Hollywood Moms

REESE WITHERSPOON

A-List Accessorizer

. . . .

Her style has shifted over the years from southern debutante (think bows, Chantilly lace, and ruffles) to a more relaxed California cool, but Reese Witherspoon has always known the importance of the small stuff—I love the way she makes simple separates pop with the addition of aviator shades, smart hats, chic scarves, denim jackets, and cute totes. Reese is also obviously a hands-on mom, which is why you'll often catch her stepping out in *normal* shoes—like metallic ballet flats or embellished sandals—when she's running errands or shuttling her kids around. (As any busy mom knows, comfy shoes are a must!)

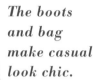

The boots and bag make casual look chic.

> *My personal style described in three words would probably be casual, simple, and lots of color.*
>
> *—Reese Witherspoon*

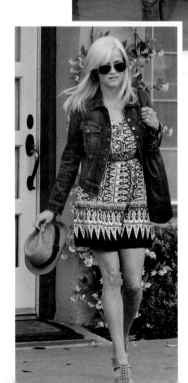

HEIDI KLUM

The Jean Queen

. . . .

From runway to red carpet, this supermodel mama is no stranger to showstopping fashions, but when Heidi Klum switches to mommy mode, she always chooses comfort over couture. And she especially loves wearing jeans: boyfriend, boot-cut, flared, and skinny styles.

While some of Klum's favorite brands include J Brand, Paige Premium Denim, and 7 for All Mankind, you really need only one great pair to steal her style. "Dark denim jeans are the essential piece to have in your closet," says stylist June Ambrose, who has worked with Kelly Ripa and Alicia Keys. "They can be worn to breakfast, lunch, or dinner, depending on what you pair them with—just make sure the hem length works with flats or heels."

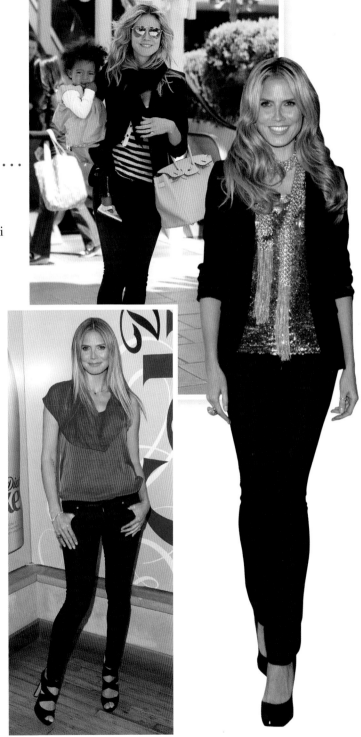

MICHELLE OBAMA

The Mix Master

. . . .

No boxy pantsuits or frumpy mom jeans here! America's First Lady of Fashion is fearless when it comes to mixing high-end couture with bargain-priced basics, and she never shies away from a bold pop of color. "She has mastered conservative with a twist," says stylist Lindsay Albanese, who has worked with celebrity moms Kendra Wilkinson and Jennifer Beals. "She's proof that it's okay to mix colors, textures, and prints that you wouldn't usually think of putting together—instead of a blue cardigan with a blue dress, she might go for a bright pink or canary yellow."

Mrs. O also has figured out what works best for her figure, so you'll see her in the same silhouette again and again. Her wardrobe essentials? Fitted cardigans in bright colors, wide belts (almost everything she wears is cinched at the waist), and one-shoulder gowns to show off her toned arms and strong shoulders. Best of all is her real-world approach to getting dressed in the morning...that's right, you will see Mrs. O wearing the same thing twice!

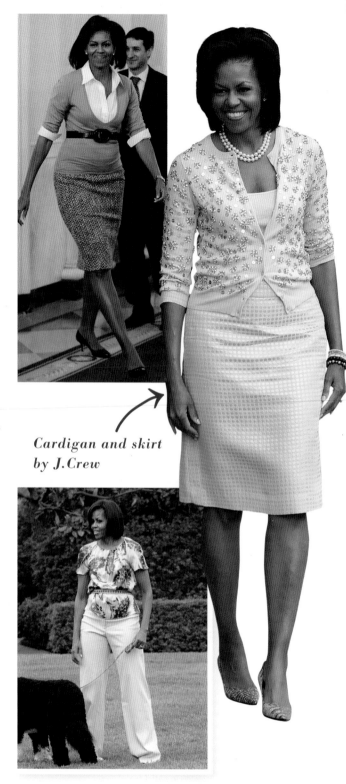

Cardigan and skirt by J.Crew

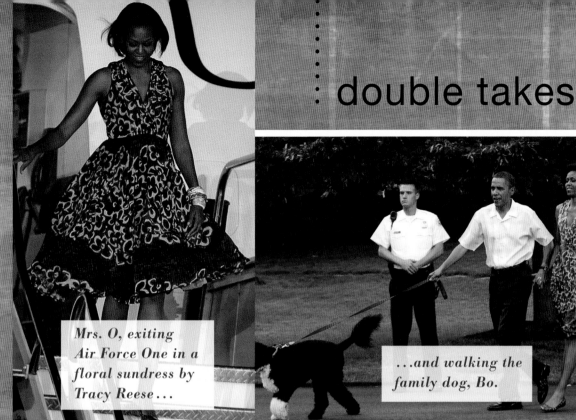

Mrs. O, exiting Air Force One in a floral sundress by Tracy Reese...

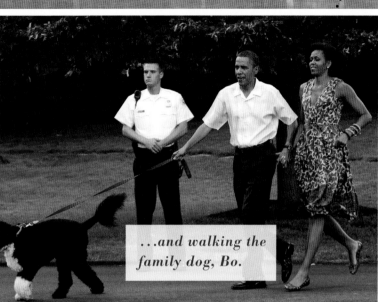

...and walking the family dog, Bo.

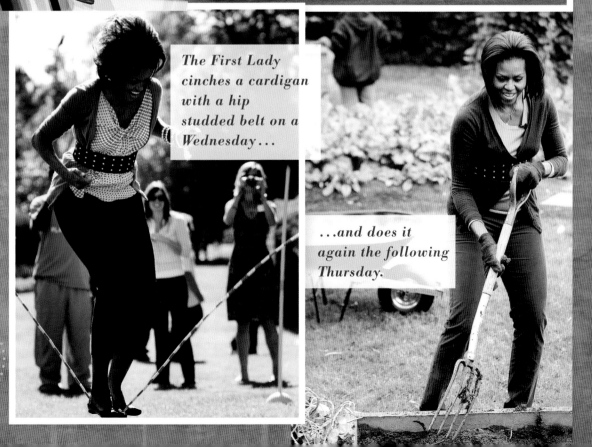

The First Lady cinches a cardigan with a hip studded belt on a Wednesday...

...and does it again the following Thursday.

ANGELINA JOLIE

The Empress of Understatement

. . . .

The globe-trotting UN goodwill
ambassador, actress, and mom of six
(Maddox, Pax, Zahara, Shiloh, Knox, and
Viv—*phew!*) sticks to fashion basics, but
never looks dowdy. Her closet is stocked
with classic pieces like pencil skirts, flat-
front pants, T-shirts, and cashmere sweaters
in a mostly neutral palette (black, beige,
and white), but she'll mix things up with an
occasional pop of red or chartreuse. The
superstar mom even keeps her Ferragamo
and Valentino accessories to a minimum,
favoring a simple black or white tote, aviator
sunglasses, and camel heels or flats. Of
course, it's hard not to look good when
you have the hottest accessory in the
world (*hello,* Brad Pitt!).

*I like to get up so every pair of
pants goes with every top, every
dress goes with every shoe. I
have a very tiny closet. Brad's
always laughing at me.*

—Angelina Jolie

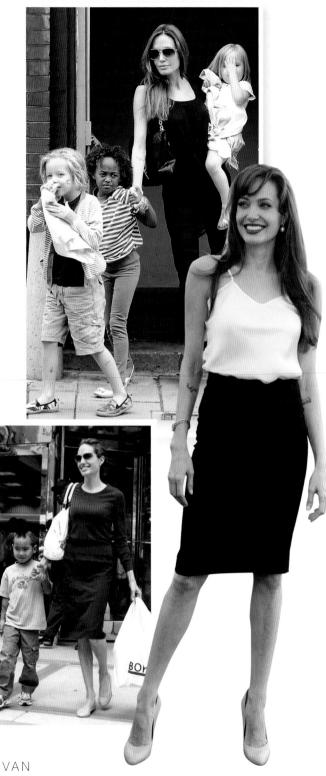

HALLE BERRY

Downtown Diva

. . . .

Since becoming a mom to daughter Nahla in 2008, this fashion risk taker hasn't lost her edge—Halle Berry is always super sexy (but never inappropriate) in cropped leather jackets, knee-high boots, and daytime dresses by Gap and BCBG Max Azria. "You rarely see her in something that's not body hugging on the red carpet, but she wears lots of flowy dresses in her downtime," says celebrity stylist Phillip Bloch, who styled the Oscar-winning actress for years. "She has that downtown edge, but she's still very feminine."

While you might want to steer clear of the head-to-toe leather look, you can still have fun with a less extreme approach. "All moms should invest in a little leather jacket to toughen up their everyday wardrobe," says Lindsay Albanese. "If black leather feels too harsh, try a softer cognac or camel shade."

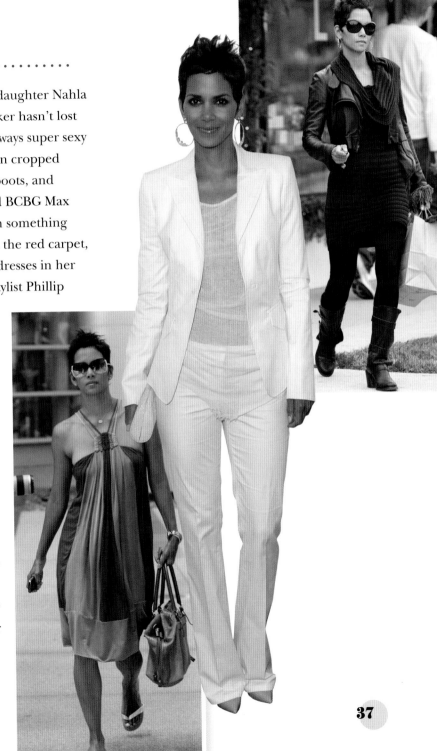

Every Mom's 10 Wardrobe Essentials

In the throws of my tenure at *Us*, I confess that I sometimes found myself obsessing over Marc Jacobs purses or contemplating which heel height was right on a pair of Christian Louboutins that I daydreamed of purchasing. Celebrity culture—and all those helpful captions identifying every last designer piece a star was wearing—made me crave things I'd never wanted or needed before, a feeling with which I'm fairly certain millions of women across the country are familiar.

Chasing trends and coveting clothes can be fun, but the truth is that it also can be a colossal waste. There was a time, for example, when those ridiculous "volume" dresses were in style, the ones that made every woman look as if she were wearing a maternity frock. I jumped on the trend late, bought up a bunch of them, and by the time I had blown more money than I care to admit, the trend was over. No woman—and certainly no mother—has the time or the money for this kind of nonsense.

The secret to effortless style is to forget the trends and build a wardrobe with basics. Don't believe me? Go back and take another peek at those best-dressed Hollywood moms. Sure, you might see a few designer handbags and some überexpensive

shoes thrown in the mix (because when you make $10 million a picture, what's a few thousand bucks?), but by and large, these chic stars keep it simple with easy-to-wear separates, a style that's easy to mimic and doesn't require breaking the bank. (In fact, more than one of those ladies has been known to shop at The Gap.)

Remember: A bubble skirt and gladiator sandals will look silly in a matter of seasons; flat-front trousers and V-neck sweaters, on the other hand, will look "current" for a lifetime. Herewith the ten essential items every mom should have in her closet. Plus, an easy tutorial on how to put all those cute basics together.

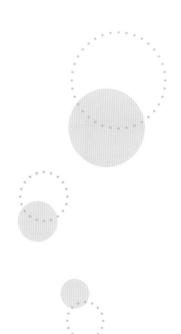

ESSENTIAL ITEM

Dark Denim

It all starts with a great pair of jeans. "Whether it's a denim trouser or a classic pair of five-pockets, a flattering pair of jeans is the style staple that you just have to have," says Lisa Axelson, the creative director responsible for Ann Taylor's recent makeover. Stick with denim in a dark all-one-color wash—you don't want details or embellishments like whiskering, holes, or rhinestones on the back pockets. For a dressier look, add a heel and a tailored blazer. On the weekend, pair denim with a fitted tee, an oversize sweater, and ballet flats for a look that's polished but still cozy. You also may want to invest in a pair of stretchy denim with Lycra, which can provide a little bit of a slimming Spanx effect (like a flatter middle and perkier tush), while also giving you some wiggle room as your weight fluctuates post-childbirth. Lycra content in denim can range anywhere from 1 to 4 percent, but choosing a 2 percent blend is best so you can avoid looking like you're wearing leggings (or worse…jeggings!).

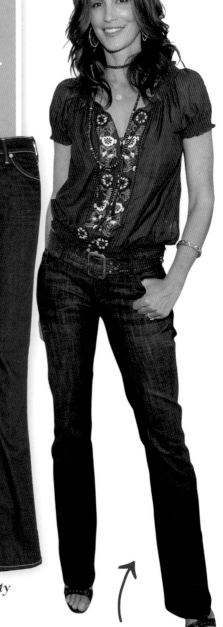

Citizens of Humanity straight-leg jeans

Celeb mom style: Cindy Crawford

ESSENTIAL ITEM

The Tunic Top

There's a reason the tunic is a perennial fashion favorite—it's not only incredibly chic, it's incredibly *forgiving*. If you've got a bit of a tummy, choose an empire style (gathered just beneath the bust). To camouflage thick thighs or a large bum, select a tunic that hits just above the knee. Whichever style you choose, try pairing the tunic with skinny jeans or leggings; slim-cut pants will counteract the full silhouette of the top.

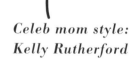

Celeb mom style: Kelly Rutherford

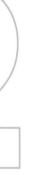

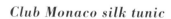

Club Monaco silk tunic

ESSENTIAL ITEM

A Classic Cardigan

. . . .

You can't go wrong when you're wearing something that's practically synonymous with style icon Jackie O. For a slightly more modern take on the classic piece, try choosing a cardigan that hits about midthigh, long enough to wear over leggings. (Keep in mind, however, that "long" is not the same as "oversized"; your cardi should still fit properly in the shoulder and sleeve, or it'll look dowdy.) A neutral color will work with everything in your closet, and it transitions easily from fall to spring. You'll also want to stick with a fine knit. Chunky cardigans are called "chunky" for a reason—they can make you look bigger.

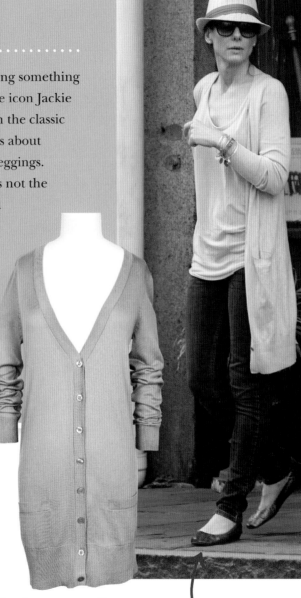

Nordstrom cardigan

Celeb mom style: Sandra Bullock

ESSENTIAL ITEM

The "Everyday" Dress

. . . .

I think women sometimes feel like dresses are a little fussy; the truth is that there's no item in your closet that's easier to wear—just throw it on and go. This sweet blue dress features a drawstring waist, which gives an otherwise roomy piece a little shape. Choose a fabric that's easy to launder—cotton is wash-and-wear simple (no wrinkles!) and will keep you cool on a sweltering summer day.

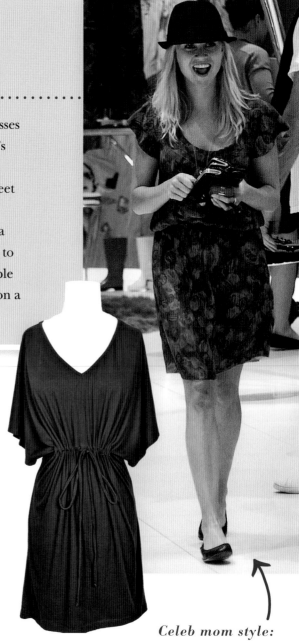

Celeb mom style: Reese Witherspoon

Simply Vera Vera Wang for Kohl's collection cotton drawstring-waist dress

ESSENTIAL ITEM

Black Leggings

· ·

Though this trend can be
supercomfortable, remember: Leggings
are not real pants. Always make sure you're
wearing them with a shirt of appropriate
length, like a tunic or an extralong
cardigan. Camel toe is a no-no!

5

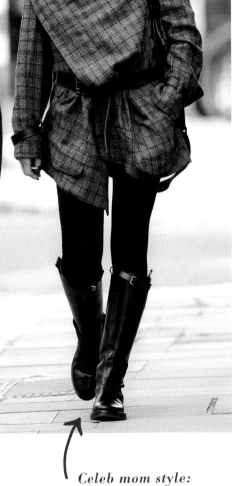

*American Apparel
cotton stretch leggings*

*Celeb mom style:
Gwen Stefani*

ESSENTIAL ITEM

The Boyfriend Jacket

. . . .

A little more fashion-forward than a blazer, the boyfriend jacket adds a bit of tomboy flair to feminine dresses and instantly adds polish when paired with dark denim. I also love the three-quarter sleeve or a jacket with sleeves that are made to be rolled up and feature a striped or white contrast lining. Make sure your jacket fits well in the shoulder but is just the slightest bit roomy through the middle.

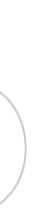

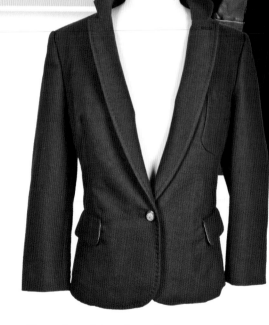

Celeb mom style:
Jessica Alba

Zara boyfriend jacket

ESSENTIAL ITEM

The Simple Shirtdress

The best thing about the shirtdress is its endless versatility. Pair it with ballet flats or espadrilles for a casual, daytime look; heels and statement jewelry make it elegant enough for evening.

7

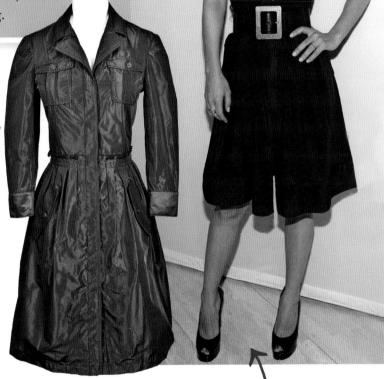

*Pink Tartan shirtdress,
Saks Fifth Avenue*

*Celeb mom style:
Giada De Laurentiis*

ESSENTIAL ITEM

A Casual Striped Tee

. . . .

Don't be afraid of a horizontal stripe—
as long as you choose a narrow pattern,
you won't look any bigger than you
actually are. Though there are a million
color combinations out there, I love a
simple stripe in navy and white, which is
reminiscent of a nautical theme
(and always, *always* in style).

8

J. Crew striped tee

Celeb mom style:
Liv Tyler

ESSENTIAL ITEM

The Fitted Pencil Skirt

. . . .

I've always found it amazing how this simple, conservatively cut skirt can look so incredibly sexy, but the key to accentuating your curves is finding a pencil with the proper fit. The length should be at or just above the knee (never below), and the width should be slim and narrow. The skirt shouldn't be so tight, however, that it curves in beneath your bum.

9

Simply Chloe Dao for QVC pencil skirt

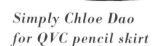

Celeb mom style: Leslie Mann

ESSENTIAL ITEM

A Wow-Worthy Red Dress

Though every woman should probably have a trusty little black dress (LBD) in her closet, don't underestimate the power of a red dress—the color is enough to make anyone feel sexy. (In fact, a study published in the *Journal of Personality and Social Psychology* found that men are most attracted to women in this color....Go figure.) Opt for a dress that's tailored or choose a wrap dress. There's a reason Diane von Furstenberg's 1970s-era invention is still so popular. It adjusts to any change in shape and is usually soft enough to hug curves in only the most flattering way. And just because a dress is red doesn't mean you can't get a lot of wear out of it. Pair it with your boyfriend jacket and you've toned it down enough for the office, while a statement necklace is all you need before a big night out.

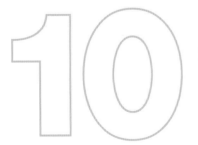

Diane von Furstenberg dress

Celeb mom style: Alessandra Ambrosio

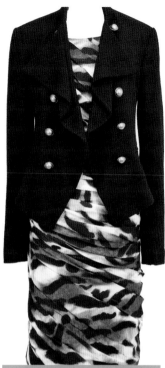

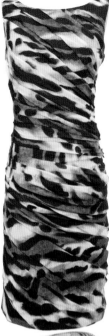

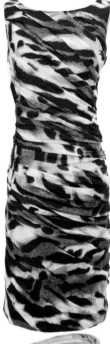

A military jacket adds oomph to a simple sheath.

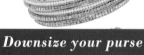

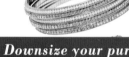

Downsize your purse or carry a small clutch.

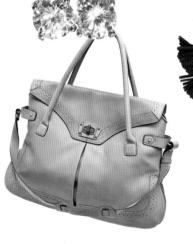

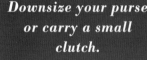

Dress, jacket, purse, and shoe by Ann Taylor

making a 9-to-5 wardrobe work 5-to-9

Lisa Axelson, Ann Taylor creative director and working mom, to the rescue

"No busy working mom has the time or the budget to shop for dual wardrobes, which is why I love the versatility of having some office-appropriate pieces that can do double duty on the weekend. For example, try dressing up distressed boyfriend jeans with a washed-silk blouse—just like the kind you'd wear to the office. Wear it untucked, and pair with ballet flats.

"To quickly take a piece of work-wear from day to evening, try swapping opaque tights for a bare or sheer leg and switching up your shoes—a high heel or a strappy sandal instantly adds sex appeal. But my favorite way to give business clothes a kick is to add dramatic jewelry. A sparkly cocktail ring or a stack of shiny bangles on your arm can easily take a daytime look from ordinary to elegant."

MIX & MATCH: SEVEN DAYS OF STYLE

Robert Verdi, E! commentator and stylist to celeb moms Ana Ortiz and Mariska Hargitay, shows how you can make your 10 Wardrobe Essentials work together.

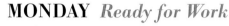

MONDAY *Ready for Work*

(Tunic top + pencil skirt)

DO wear jewelry—a sparkly earring can make you feel polished and put-together. **DO** glam up your plain pencil shirt with a sexy leopard shoe. **DON'T** pair a leopard shoe with a leopard bag; matchy-matchy accessories are old and outdated.

Quilted leather purse by Storksak doesn't look like a diaper bag but holds all the mommy essentials

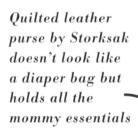

TUESDAY *Trip to the Zoo*

(Everyday dress)

DO add a little bohemian flair to an everyday dress with a long scarf. **DO** carry a diaper bag if you must, but be careful not to look like you're actually hauling diapers. Choose a chic style, like this quilted one that's smartly disguised as a purse. **DON'T** throw on sneakers with your dress!

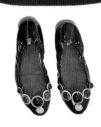

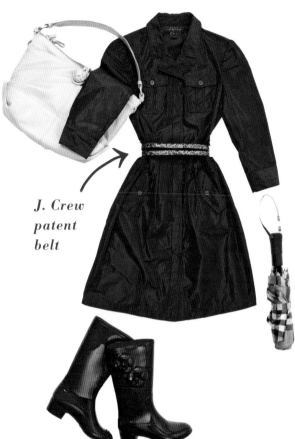

J. Crew patent belt

WEDNESDAY *PTA Meeting at School*

(Shirtdress)

DO make a fashion statement in bright rubber rain boots on a dreary day. **DO** accessorize a simple shirtdress with an unexpected belt (but **DON'T** choose one with bows or pom-poms). **DON'T** be afraid to carry a patterned umbrella.

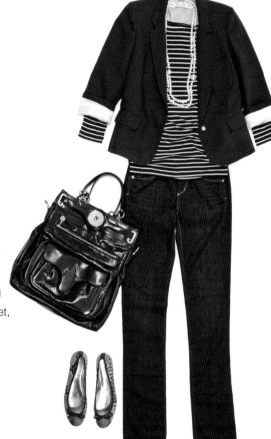

THURSDAY *Running Errands Around Town*

(Striped tee + dark denim + boyfriend jacket)

DO pair jeans with a smartly tailored jacket for a crisp, classic look. **DO** wear pearls with a casual outfit. **DON'T** wear a matching necklace, bracelet, and earrings—less is more.

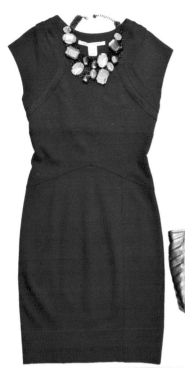

FRIDAY *Date Night*

(Red dress)

DO take a red dress from daytime to evening with a bold statement necklace. **DON'T** wear red shoes with a red dress. **DON'T** show too much leg—a red dress is sexy enough.

Zara quilted tote (under $100 and so chic—the look of Chanel or Lanvin for less!)

Banana Republic leather hobo bag

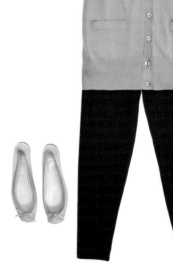

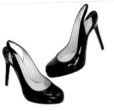

SATURDAY *Afternoon Soccer Game*

(Tunic top + cardigan + black leggings)

DO belt a long cardigan to define your waist. **DO** wear aviator shades—they look good on everyone, no matter what your face shape is. **DON'T** be afraid to layer lightweight pieces, they won't add bulk.

SUNDAY *Kids' Birthday Party*

(Shirtdress + striped tee)

DO layer a T-shirt under your dress for a more relaxed weekend look. **DO** add a pop of color with bright, feminine accessories. **DON'T** wear a fanny pack or a backpack—tote a cute canvas purse that can hold all your essentials.

J. Crew resin bead necklace (wrap it around your wrist to make a great bracelet!)

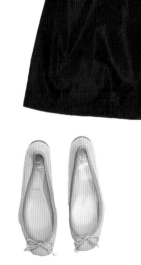

Cole Haan canvas tote

the classic trench: instant style-maker

If you're anything like I am, trying to get dressed for a last-minute dinner date or a weeknight school event is enough to trigger a mini-meltdown. Next time you're in a rush to make it out the door, take a deep breath . . . and then reach for the one style staple that's completely foolproof: the classic trench.

"The trench is endlessly versatile," says Lisa Axelson. "You can throw it on with jeans and ballet flats for that run to the grocery store, or pair it with a white shirt and trousers for a crisp, classic look." While a khaki-colored trench is timeless, don't be afraid to play with bold colors and textures—a cherry red or cheery fuchsia looks modern, and the pop of color can brighten your mood on a dreary, rainy day. "I also love the idea of a trench in an unexpected fabric, like a rainproof taffeta," adds Ken Downing, fashion director at Neiman Marcus. "It will work for inclement weather during the day and double as the perfect topper for evening."

Katie Holmes

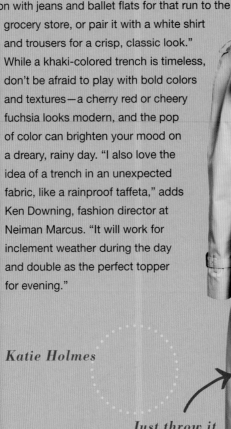

Just throw it on and go!

which shoe styles work for moms on the go?

"When you're running around town or chasing after a toddler, comfort is key—but you can find a comfortable shoe without sacrificing style," says Fred Allard, creative director at Nine West. A ballet flat is essential, but you should choose one with a little thickness to the sole (shoes that are *too* flat don't offer enough shock absorption and can actually damage the feet, hips, and knees). "When designing flats at Nine West," says Allard, "I often add a little hidden wedge for extra support." For heels, a wedge or a platform looks fashionable without being too hard to wear. In the summer months, celeb moms like Julia Roberts and Liv Tyler often step out in Toms (toms.com) or the stylishly updated clogs from Swedish shoemaker Hasbeens (available at amazon.com). And in the winter, a flat riding boot worn over jeans looks polished.

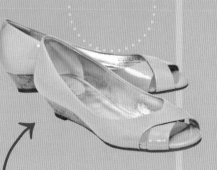

A small wedge provides support for your knees and back.

diaper bags that don't look dumpy

Q: *What's the easiest way for a new mom to look stylish and put-together?*

A: "That's easy," says Sara Blakely, owner and creator of Spanx shapewear and a new mom herself. "Invest in a diaper bag that doesn't look like a diaper bag! I didn't do that for the first two or three months after giving birth—I just used the bag that came with my breast pump. But I cannot *tell* you the difference it made when I finally went out and bought a really nice diaper bag that wasn't so dowdy. It made me feel human again!"

Take a cue from these stylish celeb moms—you'd never know their chic totes are actually filled with diapers!

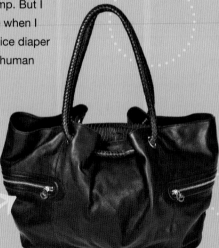

MIA BOSSI dotted "Maria" diaper bag carried by moms Jennifer Hudson and Tina Fey

JIMEALE diaper bag with matching changing mat carried by mom Isla Fisher

ROSIE POPE leather "London Shopper" bag carried by moms Nicole Richie and Jennifer Garner

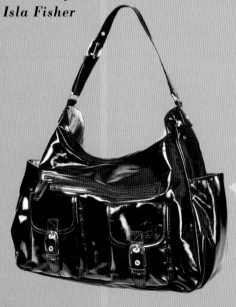

AMY MICHELLE faux patent "Sweet Pea" hobo bag carried by moms Sarah Michelle Gellar, Katherine Heigl, and Tori Spelling

QUIZ

CAN YOU GUESS WHICH COSTS LESS?

Looking stylish isn't only about money, as these look-alike steals prove.

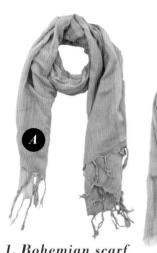
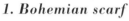
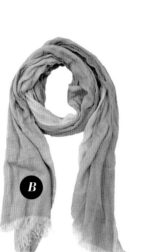

1. Bohemian scarf

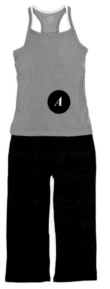
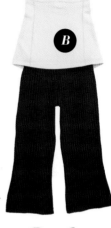

2. Casual workout wear

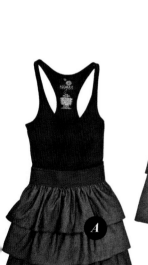
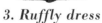

3. Ruffly dress

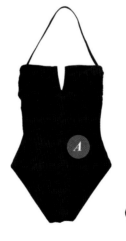
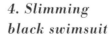

4. Slimming black swimsuit

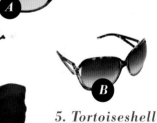

5. Tortoiseshell sunglasses

ANSWERS:

1. A: Designer label! $89, Love Quotes;
B: Knockoff! $12.50, Old Navy

2. A: Knockoff! $12.99 for the tank and $17.99 for the stretchy capris, C9 by Champion for Target; B: Designer label! $84 for the tank and $98 for the pants, Lululemon

3. A: Knockoff! $16, Miley Cyrus & Max Azria for Walmart;
B: Designer label! $295, Theory

4. A: Designer label! $425, Wolford;
B: Knockoff! $20, Norma Kamali for Walmart

5. A: Knockoff! $18, Target; B: Designer label! $325, Dior

5 ways to look thinner

1. Slim with one color Wearing different shades of a single hue (shirt, sweater, pants, and shoes) creates a continuous column of color that makes you look long and lean. Like black, shades of chocolate, wine, charcoal, and navy absorb light, so they're all excellent slenderizing options.

2. Busy patterns On the flip side, don't be afraid of bright, bold patterns. They keep the eye moving and can hide a multitude of "imperfections," as well as distract from problem parts of your body. Just keep the pattern limited to a single piece of clothing. (Meaning, don't match a brightly patterned shirt with a brightly patterned skirt.)

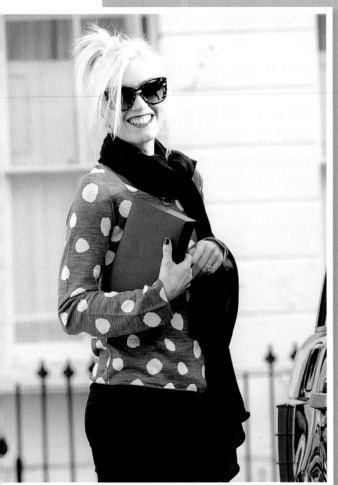

3. Statement jewelry Big earrings or a chunky necklace can draw attention away from a part of your body you might want to conceal, like a busting-out-all-over bust or a midsection that isn't as slim and trim as you'd like.

4. Try a long scarf This is another great trend started by celebrities; the long, lightweight scarf provides instant belly-bulge or awkward-boobs camouflage. It's nonseasonal, and makes even the most casual outfit look a bit more stylish and interesting.

5. Add a wide belt Cinch your middle (not too tight to avoid spillover!) in a pencil skirt. This will help you create a waist if yours is still in hiding.

How to Hide Your Jiggle in a Jiff!

Battle muffin top, belly bulge, boob droop,
and back fat with shapewear

From the rolls that spill over the top of your jeans (muffin top) to those unsightly bulges above and below the bra band (otherwise known as back fat), that extra jiggle around the middle is one of the lingering gifts of pregnancy. Even if you do get back down to your pre-pregnancy weight, it's entirely possible that some of that fat will remain redistributed in places it wasn't before. While a healthy diet and regular exercise can *help* (and should certainly be part of your postpartum routine), the fastest way to put your slimmest self forward is to give your wardrobe a tweak. Here's how to look svelte—even when you feel like a sausage.

DON'T STUFF YOURSELF INTO TOO-TIGHT CLOTHING

Lots of new moms try to squeeze into clothes that don't flatter their figure, just because they're terrified of going up a dress size. "It's a psychological thing," says Sara Blakely. "Women want to do everything *but* go up a size. The irony is that you'll look better if you do. I decided to let it go after I gave birth—if looking great meant buying a dress a size or two larger, then fine." In other words, you're not fooling anyone by wearing clothes that just don't fit. In fact, too-tight clothing most likely will make you appear heavier.

DITCH THE CLINGY T-SHIRTS

You'll want to avoid wearing tees and sweaters that cling to the body—especially for the first few months after delivery—but you also don't want to wear big boxy shirts that don't have any shape. The compromise? Tops that are gathered at the bust and slightly loose at the bottom. "Since your chest is bigger after giving birth, you can play up that part of your body to distract from the tummy," says Blakely. "Of course, I'm not suggesting you reveal massive amounts of cleavage. Just look for shirts that come in under the chest, like an empire-style top."

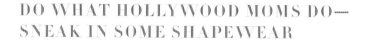

DO WHAT HOLLYWOOD MOMS DO— SNEAK IN SOME SHAPEWEAR

Thanks largely to the monumental success of Spanx, the subject of jiggle-controlling compression panties is no longer taboo. Even Gwyneth Paltrow admitted to wearing two pairs of Spanx (at the same time!) after the birth of her daughter, Apple—and women everywhere breathed a massive sigh of relief. "When a beautiful woman that we all look at and admire admits to getting a little help from a supportive undergarment, we know we're not alone," says Spanx's Blakely.

A high-waisted compression garment that stops just below the bra band will smooth out any lumps and bumps and can be worn under practically anything, from dresses to skirts to jeans or even shorts. "Just don't wear anything that cuts you in half or that stops around the belly button," says Blakely. "You don't want to create a ring of fat around your middle."

I'm always wearing Spanx. I wear Spanx to bed. My husband is like, What is this on you? And I say, Trust me, it's better. Everything is better in Spanx!

—*Actress and mom of three*
JULIE BOWEN

how to select the right shapewear

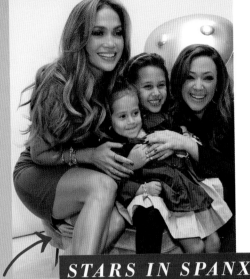

It's no secret that celebrities have been raving about the slimming magic of Spanx for a few years now (usually it's because they're attending so many fabulous events, like the Oscars, the Emmys, and the Golden Globes, and they have to wear slinky gowns in front of photographers). Since most of us, ahem, *regular* women don't usually have occasion to suck ourselves into an Herve Leger dress and pose on the red carpet, I think we got the impression that shapewear wasn't created with us in mind or that it's too confining to wear every day. So not true! The market for slimming and smoothing panties has exploded, so you'll easily find comfortable undies you can wear every day, as well as full-body shapers for those nights when you want to pour yourself into an elegant LBD. A simple piece of shapewear can give you the confidence to get back in the clothes you loved pre-pregnancy—and that's why *every* mom should have some in her closet.

STARS IN SPANX

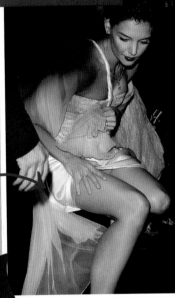

For EVERYDAY coverage

Spanx Undie-tectable Panty, a great tummy-taming option when you don't want to wear a shaper that comes all the way up to the bra band. Perfect under shorts and jeans.

Spanx Skinny Britches are a lightweight and supersheer option when you need more comfy coverage.

For MEDIUM coverage

Spanx Skinny Britches Short, a longer version of the Skinny Britches undies, are ultralight and designed for layering—wear one to slim, two to shape, and three when you really want to suck it in.

Assets Mid-Thigh Shaper from Spanx's more budget-friendly sister line (available at Target) features a leg-band-free design, smoothing the tummy, thighs, and bum without bulging. Fantastic under skirts.

Assets Fantastic Firmers Tank eliminates tummy bulge, muffin top, and back fat, and you can wear it under everything.

For MAXIMUM coverage

Spanx In-Power Line Super Higher Power is a super high-waisted, midthigh shaper with a seriously slimming tummy control panel. "Megacompression" zones minimize love handles, lift your bum, and give you an hourglass shape, all without VPL (visible panty lines).

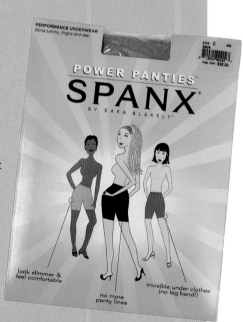

PERFORMANCE UNDERWEAR
Slims tummy, thighs and rear.

size: C

POWER PANTIES
SPANX
BY SARA BLAKELY

look slimmer & feel comfortable

no more panty lines

invisible under clothes (no leg band!)

BATTLING THE BOOB DROOP AND BACK FAT

From pregnancy to breastfeeding and beyond, your bust size has undoubtedly changed, especially if you're still shedding those last few pounds of baby weight. Not only can the right bra create a slimming effect under your clothes, but—as we discussed in chapter 1—it can save you from a case of permanent boob droop. Here's what you need to know about getting a bra that really fits.

Don't Be a Slave to Size

While it's important to know your measurements (and to get remeasured every so often, since the size of your breasts will undoubtedly change over time), don't disregard the way a bra looks and—more important—*feels* when you try it on. "One of the biggest mistakes that women make is getting it stuck in their minds that they can only wear a particular size," says Spanx's Blakely. "Don't think that you're a 34B just because you've been a 34B since high school."

When you head to the dressing room, take the time to try on a bra one size smaller and one size bigger than what you're used to wearing. "I've never actually worn the bra size that I measured for," says Blakely.

"When I'm wearing the size I'm supposed to be wearing, I feel bound across my rib cage." Instead, go for comfort—the right bra shouldn't pinch under the arms or across the back.

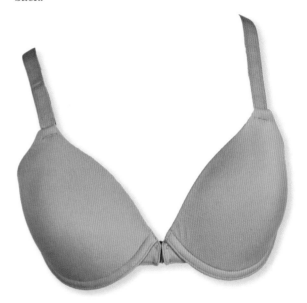

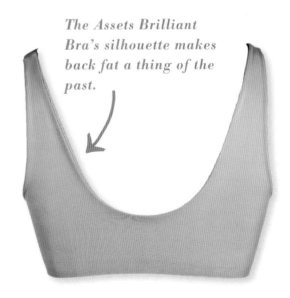

The Assets Brilliant Bra's silhouette makes back fat a thing of the past.

Don't Forget Your Back!

"Women often focus only on how they look in a bra from the front," says Blakely. "But it's important to inspect the fit from the front *and* the back." A bra that's too tight will cause underarm bulge, that spillage of fat between your boob and your armpit, and will pinch across the back (and create lumps and bumps under your clothes). When you're satisfied with the bra itself, put your shirt back on and see how it looks. "You should choose a cup that gives your chest a smooth look under T-shirts," says Blakely. That means no gaping, no poking, no pinching, and no bumpy lace showing through.

For a seriously smooth look, Spanx makes the Bra-llelujah!, an all-hosiery bra with no hooks, wires, clasps, or bulges (Debra Messing and Jennifer Garner are fans), as well as the lower-priced Assets Brilliant Bra. "I love them because they lie flat on your back and are smooth under T-shirts," says Blakely. "They don't create all that bulge, that back fat hanging everywhere."

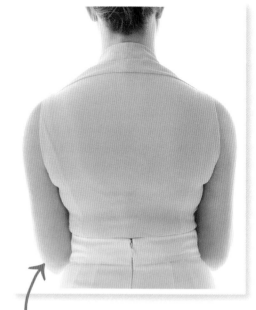

The wrong bra will pinch and add bulk...

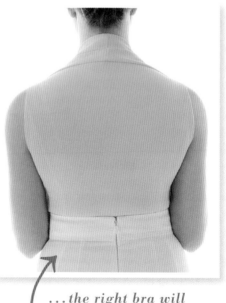

...the right bra will look sleek and smooth under clothes.

Swimsuit Shopping 101

When my husband and I were preparing to move our family from New York to Los Angeles in 2010 (and packing up our apartment), I came across some photos from our honeymoon in Hawaii. I was only twenty-eight then, but I never really loved my body; I was always wishing I were taller, fitter, thinner, and always felt self-conscious in a bikini. But there I was on the beach, prancing around in a two-piece, and boy, what I wouldn't give to go back in time and smack some sense into myself. I looked great back then! (Writer Nora Ephron once said, "Oh, how I regret not having worn a bikini the entire time I was twenty-six.") And I'm glad there's some photographic evidence to prove that, at some point in my life, I had the vague outline—the near promise—of a six-pack (instead of the minikeg that most of us moms carry around). These days, I wouldn't be caught dead in a bikini.

"The whole concept of wearing a swimsuit is kind of crazy," admits swimwear designer and mom Shoshanna Gruss, whose cute suits have been worn by celeb moms like Britney Spears and Selma Blair. "It's basically like walking out of the house in your underwear." But let's face it, unless you want to be that weird mom in a muumuu who never gets wet, squeezing into a suit is unavoidable. There are ways, however, to make the process less painful. After all, if you've actually managed to schedule a blissfully relaxing day at the beach (or even if you're just spending another sunny afternoon at the neighborhood pool), the last thing on your mind should be your suit.

WHAT IF I DON'T EVEN KNOW WHERE TO START?

If you've only recently become a mom—or you just haven't had the courage to shop for a swimsuit in a while—there is some good news. In the last few years, swimwear companies finally have figured out that not all women are a cookie-cutter size. Every day there are more and better styles designed with different body issues in mind. For example, you can find suits with hidden control panels and Miracle Bra technology (or padding on the bust that doesn't look totally fake). The shapewear brands Spanx and Maidenform Control It! offer their own suck-you-in swimwear. Even Speedo sells a line of suits with "360° Core Control." "When I first started designing swimwear, no one was selling tops and bottoms as separates," says Gruss. "But my line offers thirteen different sizes, since a woman may feel great about her top and not her bottom, or vice versa."

When you do go shopping, it's also a good idea to prepare the way you would before heading to the beach: Shave your legs, get groomed, and apply self-tanner. "Dressing rooms are depressing," says Gruss. "The lighting is awful, and who wants to take their clothes off only to feel terrible about themselves? You want to look and feel as good as you can when you go in there."

CAN I REALLY BUY A SWIMSUIT ONLINE?

Yes, especially if it's photographed well. "Many women can get a feel for whether or not a suit will flatter their figure just by seeing it first on a body or a dress form," says Gruss. "That's harder to do when a suit is just hanging on a rack." The other obvious benefit of shopping online is that you can try on swimsuits in the privacy of your own home—many companies now offer free shipping and returns, so you can order several sizes without putting a strain on your wallet.

WHEN IS IT TIME TO SWITCH TO A ONE-PIECE?

Becoming a mom doesn't necessarily mean you have to switch up your swimwear. Looking cute on the beach is more about comfort and confidence than it is about wearing a particular style. "I'm a mom and I still wear a string bikini," says Gruss. "But I definitely have a newfound appreciation for one-pieces. They can be really sexy. Plus, I can run around with my daughter without having to check and make sure that everything's still inside my suit!"

So how old is too old to wear a bikini? "I don't like to put an exact number on it," says Gruss. "There are some young women who are overweight and out of

A loose-fitting tankini is the most flattering.

shape, just like there are women in their fifties and sixties who work out every day and have incredible figures. But if you're getting a lot of strange looks, it might be time to switch styles." For a great middle-of-the-road option, try the tankini—you can pull it up while you're sunbathing or pull it down to cover your tummy while you're walking around. For the most flattering silhouette, choose a style that's fitted under the bust and loose around the middle.

WHICH STYLES ARE BEST FOR A BIGGER BUST?

You'll need a suit with adequate support and construction, which you're more likely to find in brands that build and size their suits like bras (go online and check out Athleta, which is owned by The Gap). "We offer sizes A through DDD, plus a few sizes within each size," says Gruss of her eponymous line. "Each woman's body is so unique, it doesn't make sense that everyone would fit into a small, medium, or large."

A bra top is a great choice for women with larger chests—it's a cute retro shape, but it's got the added support of an underwire. If you're not a fan of boning or wire in your swimwear, opt for a halter style

instead. "Halters typically have a wide band underneath the bust to help hold you up," says Gruss. Even the teeny bandeau can be an option, if you find one that's built like a real strapless bra. "Lots of women think they can't wear a bandeau because it usually fits like a tube," says Gruss. "The key is to find one with hidden support."

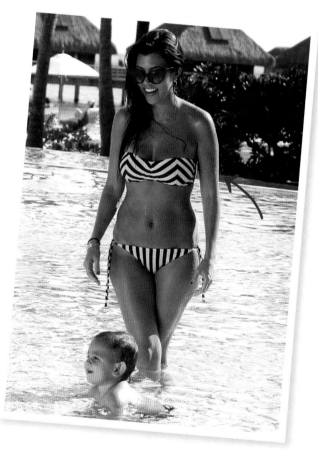

Mom Kourtney Kardashian in a bandeau that's built to give support.

HOW CAN I DOWNPLAY THE TUMMY AREA?

One word: ruching! Even a well-cut one-piece can be tight in the middle, drawing attention to the lumps, bumps, and cellulite that you don't want to show. Ruching, however, is perfect for camouflaging a little belly bulge because it doesn't give you that same skintight look. Best of all, ruching is a beautiful fashion detail, so it doesn't necessarily make you look like you're trying to hide something.

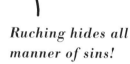

Ruching hides all manner of sins!

BESIDES BLACK, WHAT COLORS ARE MOST SLIMMING?

You don't have to wear a matronly black one-piece to look slim on the beach. "Deep colors, like a dark purple, as well as prints in dark tones are all good choices," says Gruss. "But looking trim is really less about the color and more about the cut. Even if you have a great figure, an ill-fitting suit just doesn't look good." When you're trying on swimwear, wiggle around a bit in the dressing room to make sure you can move comfortably without falling out. (Remember, you're going to be running around after your kids in this thing.) And just like lingerie, a swimsuit shouldn't be too loose, but it also shouldn't be digging into your skin.

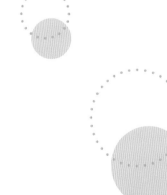

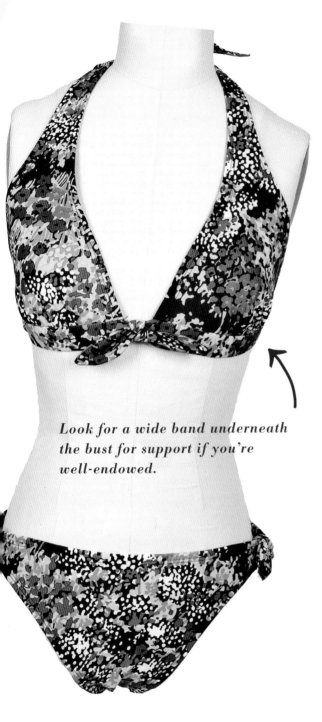

Look for a wide band underneath the bust for support if you're well-endowed.

ARE THERE CERTAIN STYLES THAT MOMS SHOULD AVOID?

"The boy short—it cuts women in a funny place, making their legs look shorter and their thighs look bigger," says Gruss. "There's just nothing appealing or sexy about that." Instead, opt for a high-cut or V-cut bottom, which will elongate the legs and give you a prettier line. If you're not totally comfortable baring your backside, you can always tie on a wrap or a sheer sarong for added coverage.

High-waisted bikini bottoms also have come back into fashion, but beware: If you're not in pretty great shape, this retro style can come off as matronly. Steer clear if you've got a tummy pooch.

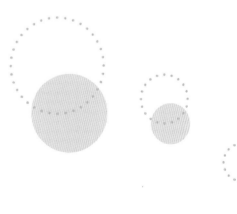

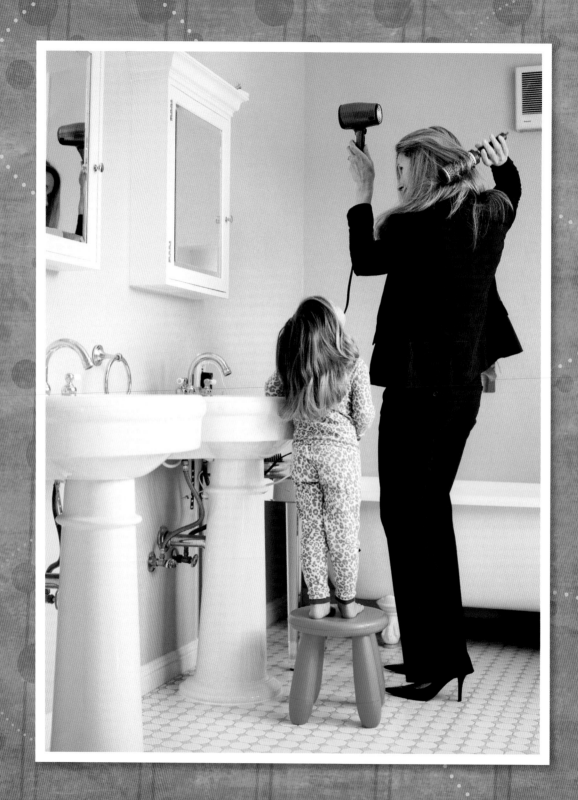

hair that looks like you care

Avoiding the Top Hair Mistakes That Frazzled Moms Make

Does any woman actually, *truly*, love her hair? It seems to me that every single female in the world has a fantasy of swapping locks with someone. Straight-haired ladies slave over curling irons and round brushes to add body and waves, while wavy- and curly-haired women religiously straighten their tresses with flat irons, Brazilian blowouts, and expensive salon visits. Brunettes want to be blond, blondes want to be brunette, and everyone feels some kind of vague pressure that, whatever they are doing to their hair, it simply is *not enough*. "My hair would be so much better if only I…[fill in the blank]."

I have been down the rabbit hole of hair insecurity many, many times. My bathroom drawers are stuffed with hot rollers, Velcro rollers, multiple curling irons, two different flat irons (because I just *had* to have a travel-size one), gels, mousses, pomades, waxes, volumizers, hair sunscreens, and glossing sprays. I think some of these products, many of which hardly have been used, are nearing their tenth anniversary of living in my bathroom. Then there is the stuff that happens at the salon. Once my regular hairstylist at a well-known salon in New York started wondering aloud why I didn't have highlights in my hair. The thought had never crossed my mind. But he asked in such a way that I felt as if I was somehow missing out on some vital part of the female experience, as if *everyone* had highlights, and somehow my invitation to the party had been lost in the mail. So I succumbed, and then every six weeks or so, I had to go back and do it again. And again. A few months later, I'd had enough. Highlights were exhausting and expensive. And that was even before I had kids.

Still, our hair does matter. Perhaps more than any other physical attribute, it sends an instant message about who we are, and it makes a lasting impression. Moms with chronically disheveled strands tell the world they're harried and barely holding on. A woman with a short, curled-under pouf may convey maternal competence, but she's no one you'd necessarily want to go shopping with. The PTA president who's the first to bake cookies but the last to cover her roots makes it known that she's at the bottom of her totem pole. And an überfrosted reverse mullet (*hello*, Kate Gosselin circa 2009) reveals there's a lioness roaming suburbia.

Of course, maintaining your mane gets a little more complicated when you factor in all the ways our hair changes after having children. Fluctuations in estrogen—during and after pregnancy—can affect not only your hair's length (since, as discussed in chapter 1, estrogen prolongs the hair's growth phase), but also its look, shape, and texture; stick-straight hair might develop a little wave, or naturally wavy hair might transition into corkscrew curls. (You may have caught a glimpse of these types of changes during puberty—another time when our hormones go haywire.) Likewise, your hair may appear thinner and finer as you enter menopause and your estrogen levels start to plummet. In fact, the condition of your hair might even change from week to week, depending on where you are in the menstrual cycle (when you're PMSing, for example, you might notice that your hair appears a little oilier).

Luckily, getting gorgeous locks—or at least having hair that looks like you care—doesn't have to mean spending hours at the salon; overdone, overfried hair is not only old-school, it makes you look old. (No one has time for that kind of primping, anyway.) In fact, the newer way to appear polished and put-together is to sport a carefree mane that looks just a little *un*done, and doesn't take thirty minutes to style. Consider this: During my first salon visit after moving to L.A., my brand-new stylist appeared hypercritical of my just-below-the-chin style. He said it was too layered, too hard to do, and then he asked how it looked if I let it air dry. Terrible, I told him. He did not mince words: "Then it doesn't work. We must change it." And after just a few appointments, he had whipped my tresses into shape. My hair was longer, with fewer layers, and—for the first time in my life—I had a cut that was truly versatile. I could let it air dry, or spend just a few minutes styling it. It could even be swept back into a no-fuss ponytail. Discovering your own easy-to-manage style—which this chapter will help you to do—means you've got one less thing to stress about in the morning. And you might just turn some heads in the process.

does your haircut make the cut?

A quality haircut should not only look good, it should be easy to maintain. It may be time to pay a visit to the salon if...

* *Your hair takes too long to style* You should be able to make it out the door in about fifteen minutes. "If you're laboring in vain for half an hour, you're in trouble," says famed NYC colorist Louis Licari.

* *You need more product than a beauty school* More isn't always more—the days of using multiple sprays, balms, and fixatives are gone. You should need only one or two products, tops, to get your hair looking good.

* *Your arm is falling off from using multiple electronics*—and I'm not talking about iPads or cell phones. Your daily routine shouldn't call for more than one appliance.

* *Your hair falls flat by ten A.M.* "A good cut should look good all day long," says Licari. If you're looking flat and frizzy by midmorning, get another cut (or a new stylist).

* *You have to pile on the makeup* Makeup is an accessory designed to aid your look; it shouldn't steal the show. If you're using glamorous earrings or pounds of bronzer and eye shadow to compensate for ho-hum hair, it's time to update your 'do.

are you making these mom-hair mistakes?

The Overfried and Overdyed

Long, crinkly, overprocessed hair with split ends screams, "I've given up!" How to fix it? "Put yourself on a schedule and get your hair cut regularly," says Licari, who has worked with stars such as Susan Sarandon, Scarlett Johansson, Katie Couric, and Michelle Pfeiffer. Try making an appointment for your next cut before checking out of the salon (even though I know that's not always realistic). To keep your hair healthy between appointments, switch to a sulfate-free shampoo (they're gentler on color-treated hair), deep condition once a week (try Bumble and bumble deeep), or try using a dab of Moroccan oil to moisturize and tame flyaways.

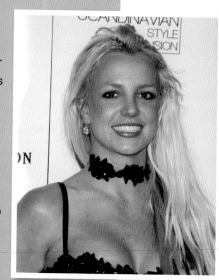

The Mullet

Kate Gosselin's asymmetrical/Florence Henderson/reverse mullet wedge of 2009 may go down in history as iconic, but for all the wrong reasons. "Business in the front and party in the back," says Licari. "You just can't pull that off." It's best not to expect your haircut to multitask.

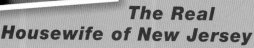

The Real Housewife of New Jersey

Do people see your big hair coming before they see you? Does no one want to sit behind you at the movies? If you have to freeze your hair into place before heading out (or if you could pass for an extra in a Whitesnake video), think twice before picking up that aerosol can. "Poufy, excessively coiffed hairstyles are old-fashioned," says Licari.

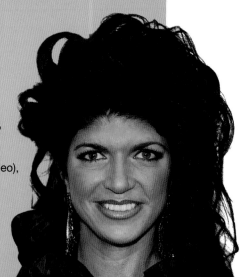

5 Easy Cuts

Since lots of busy mothers tend to think of basic beauty maintenance and regular salon appointments as unnecessary luxuries, it's easy to find yourself stuck in a years-long hair rut. Getting trimmed regularly, however, can actually *save* you time over the long term. Dry, damaged hair and split ends make for more difficult styling, create more frizzies and flyaways, and generally require more product to tame (leaving you with a 'do that looks greasy, crunchy, and gross). If you can swing it, consider splurging on a quality cut at a more expensive salon to get the basic shape right and having it trimmed every eight to twelve weeks by a more budget-friendly stylist—you'll maintain that just-stepped-out-of-the-salon look without spending a fortune.

THE LIBERTY

This long, layered look—so named for its carefree, wash-and-wear quality—comes courtesy of celebrity hairstylist Oscar Blandi. It's "leave-it-alone hair because it's so easy to style," he says. (He also calls it "the Kelly Ripa.") The cut is almost universally flattering and works with most textures. If your strands are fine and straight, stick with a length no longer than your collarbone. For wavy or curly hair, you'll need fewer layers.

**WORKS
BEST FOR:
*All hair types***

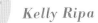

Kelly Ripa

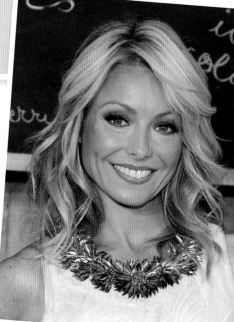

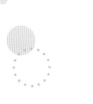

THE CLASSIC BOB

. . . .

This chic style conveys sophistication without much fuss, transitioning effortlessly from nine-to-five to overtime. (It's also helped clean up the image of many a Hollywood mom—think Christina Aguilera in one of her many earlier incarnations.) The only catch? Make sure it doesn't flip at the ends, or you'll wind up with the dreaded "mom hair." Personally, I tried to emulate the sleek Katie Holmes–style bob of 2007, but with the slightest ounce of humidity it would pouf up and become round. I resembled a bobblehead, so I grew it out.

To avoid such embarrassing blunders, celeb stylist Dominick Pucciarello, who has worked with A-list moms Sarah Jessica Parker, Heidi Klum, Gisele Bündchen, and Candice Bergen, recommends going with a stick-straight blowout (if you can manage that on your own) or flipping your head over and spritzing with hair spray for a messed-up, rock 'n' roll look. Adding subtle layers can also help prevent unwanted pouf.

WORKS BEST FOR:
Medium to fine hair; a blunt edge will make fine hair appear thicker.

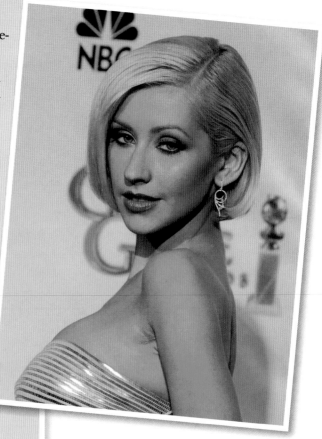

Christina Aguilera

THE LONG BOB

A cut that's a bit below the chin with angled layers or bangs is the quickest way to slim down and help define a round face. Plus, this look is supersimple to maintain and very forgiving during those first few months post-pregnancy. "Aim for something that's just above shoulder length, with graduated layers around the face and about one inch from the bottom," says Blandi. "Once the hairs start to split on the shoulder, it's time for a trim."

WORKS BEST FOR:
All hair types

THE FRINGE

Lots of new moms experience some hair loss within a few months of giving birth (sprouting a little horseshoe of baby hairs at the hairline is also common), but bangs can create a sense of fullness, camouflage a high forehead, and even cover wrinkles and worry lines. In fact—short of Botox injections—a side-swept fringe paired with layered hair is the fastest way to shave years off your look (see next page). To help draw attention to the eyes and cheekbones, ask your stylist to add in some layers at midcheek. "They'll lift the face right up, as well as create some swing and movement," says Licari.

WORKS BEST FOR:
Hair that's naturally straight or wavy, not curly

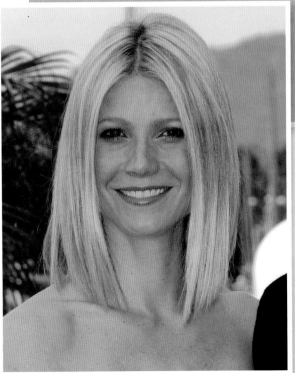

Gwyneth Paltrow

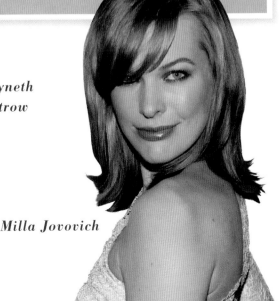

Milla Jovovich

take off 5 years...with bangs!

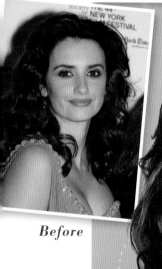

Before

After

Michelle Obama

What works Obama's fringe conceals lines on her forehead, says hairstylist Charles Baker Strahan, who has worked with celebrity moms Mariah Carey and Gretchen Mol. And lustrous bangs reflect light, enhancing her glow and shaving years off her face.

What to avoid A stiff style (like her "before" photo) gives her a matronly, helmet-head look. Bangs and layers add movement, says Ricardo Rojas, who has styled Heidi Klum.

Penélope Cruz

What works A side-swept bang, paired with long layers that start below the chin, can downplay a square jaw, says stylist Kim Vo, who has worked with Kate Hudson and Jenny McCarthy.

What to avoid Big hair that's slicked back can make a square face appear boxy. Same goes for blunt-cut, Dutch-boy bangs.

Before

After

THE PIXIE

This cut may seem somewhat boyish, but there's nothing masculine about it when styled correctly. (Blandi calls this look "the gamine.") Unlike the punk 'dos of the 1980s, the latest incarnation is softer, with sexy pieces around the face to maximize the cheekbones, eyes, and jaw. Since the pixie is a cropped look, it requires a trim every six to eight weeks, but it's practically wash-and-wear simple.

What you *don't* want: Anything too cropped, shaved in the back, or that has sideburns. (If you've been called "sir" from someone standing behind you, you've got to grow it out.) Licari warns that this style *can* look a bit severe on older women (since as we age, our faces tend to lose their softness), and it's best suited for those with delicate features. As someone who's had this haircut before, I know that the pixie can make you look a little mannish unless you're slight in frame and might require chic, feminine little outfits to maximize that gamine look.

WORKS BEST FOR:
Medium to fine hair; thick, coarse hair might frizz too easily

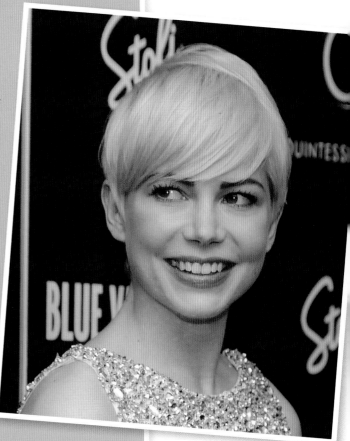

Michelle Williams

Fast Hair Fixes When You Have No Time

Not every mom has an hour to luxuriate in the shower and give herself a leisurely blowout before getting the kiddos off to school. (Actually, I don't know *any* mother who has that kind of time in the morning—or ever.) Instead of whisking back your hair in an unstylish scrunchie or sporting an embarrassing case of bed head, try one of these mini mom-hair makeovers the next time you're running a bit behind schedule—they'll help get you out the door *fast*, without sacrificing an ounce of style.

MOM MISTAKE
Greasy Tresses

You know the feeling: It's your morning to carpool, but you've overslept, you're simultaneously whipping up a PB&J for your daughter's lunch box while attempting to locate her missing shoes, and you're trying to make it out the door in the next three and a half minutes. A quick glance in the mirror reveals yet another problem— your unwashed hair resembles an oil slick. No time to shower? No problem.

5-MINUTE FIX
Dry Shampoo

If you haven't already picked yourself up a bottle of this miracle product, drop everything. Dry shampoo (most often sold in an aerosol can) absorbs oil, eliminates odor, adds volume and lift, and makes your hair look and feel clean, no water necessary. Whether you've loaded too much product on your hair or just haven't washed it, a quick spray will make it *appear* as though your personal hygiene is still a priority. My favorites are Klorane Gentle Dry Shampoo with Oat Milk and Oscar Blandi Pronto Dry Shampoo Spray (both available at sephora.com). For a tinted version—which can help cover up gray—try Bumble and bumble Hair Powder (available in four shades; bumbleandbumble.com) or Orlando Pita T3 Refresh Volumizing Dry Shampoo (available in three shades; sephora.com).

MOM MISTAKE
The Butterfly Clip

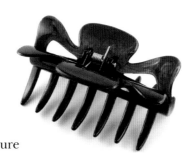

It may be a foolproof way to keep flyaways off your face, but the butterfly clip is dated and dowdy, a sure sign that perhaps you never outgrew those sorority house slumber parties.

5-MINUTE FIX
The LBH (Little Black Headband)

This easy-to-wear staple has made a *major* comeback—Hollywood moms like Jessica Alba and Gwyneth Paltrow sport them everywhere from the playground to the red carpet. Avoid looking like a member of the Junior League by choosing a headband that's very thin and very plain. Black is best, though a little sparkle works well for evening (but no bows!). *Access Hollywood*'s Maria Menounos is a fan of the bands by ban.dō (available at shopbando.com).

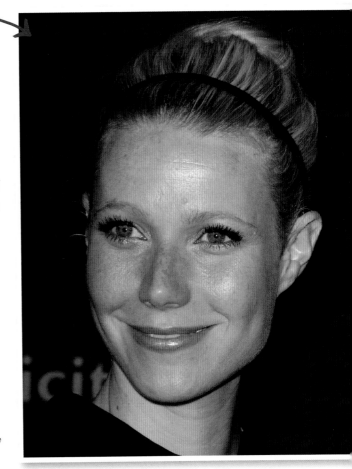

Gwyneth Paltrow

MOM MISTAKE
Visible Grays

You're between salon appointments and a number of grays have sprouted along the hairline, or you've started to notice your first not-so-subtle signs of aging and haven't had time to buy that box of just-right color or track down an expert colorist.

Jennifer Lopez

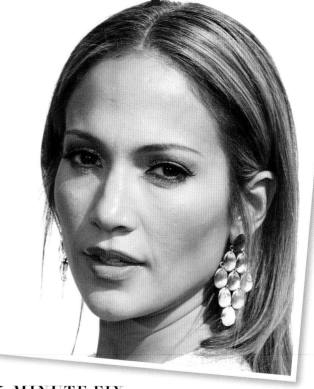

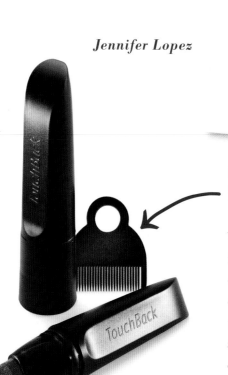

5-MINUTE FIX
Temporary Hair Marker

While a number of hair care brands, including L'Oréal, Clairol, and Revlon, offer root touch-up kits that make at-home color correction a breeze, the fastest way to erase errant grays is with TouchBack, a temporary hair color marker that deposits color until your next shampoo. It contains no harsh chemicals, and it won't rub or flake off. Genius! (Available at touchbackgray.com.)

MOM MISTAKE
The Scrunchie

The fabric-covered ponytail holder went out with glossy tights and Aerobicise videos… *on VHS*. If you're still using a poufy, patterned scrunchie to whisk the hair back against the nape of your neck, it's time for an update.

5-MINUTE FIX
The Chic Pony

While it's true that lots of busy moms are overreliant on the ponytail (including me), it *is* possible to create a look that's a little sleeker. Start by sectioning the hair at the top of your head and then back-combing ever so lightly with your fingers or a teasing comb. Spritz a little root-lift spray at the crown, smooth down the sides, and pull back the hair with a plain elastic band (one that matches your hair color). "This way you get some lift at the crown, so your hair doesn't look flat and frumpy," says celeb hairstylist Tippi Shorter. "It's a polished look that you can wear out at night, too."

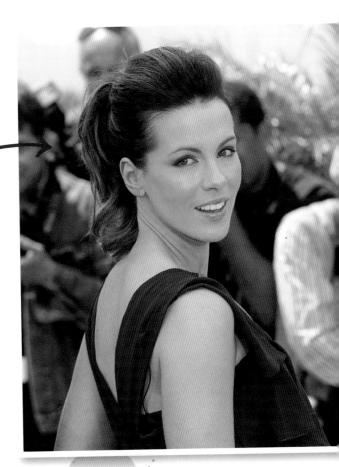

Kate Beckinsale

when all else fails—hide it under a hat!

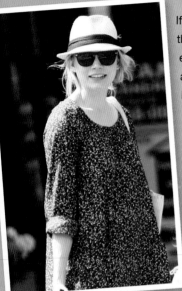

If you're having the bad hair day to end all bad hair days—and we've all been there—a stylish hat can disguise the dilemma, keep the sun off your skin, and even add oomph to an outfit. (In fact, your girlfriends may think you spent *hours* agonizing over what to wear.) Here's how to pull off the chicest caps without looking like you've got something to hide.

The Straw Fedora

How to wear it Choose a fedora with a flat brim that's not too wide; the hat itself should sit relatively low over your eyes, not high up on the head.

Pair it with A casual summer dress and flats or dark denim and a classic cardigan.

The Slouchy Knit Hat

How to wear it The style looks best when you allow a few tresses to escape from underneath it; stuffing all your hair in the cap can look too severe, as well as make the face appear rounder. Pull the hat back an inch or two from the hairline (it shouldn't sit low over the eyes), and finger sweep your bangs or face-framing layers forward.

Pair it with Since the hat itself is casual, it looks best when paired with clothing that's a little more put-together, like jeans and a khaki trench or a sleek overcoat.

Michelle Williams

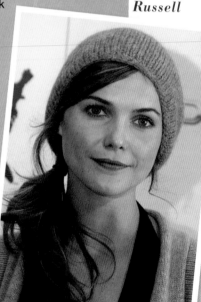

Keri Russell

The Driving Cap or Newsboy

How to wear it Whether patterned or plain, this cap should be worn with the brim flat and pulled down low on the forehead.

Pair it with The driving cap—potentially the trickiest style to pull off—can look a little awkward with mountains of hair billowing out from underneath it. Try pulling the hair back in a messy bun and donning a chic pair of sunglasses for effortless-looking style.

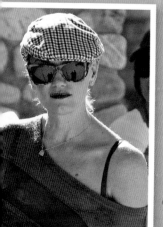

Gwen Stefani

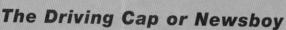

To Color or Not to Color?

Somewhere around age thirty, most of us notice that our hair gradually starts to dull and fade. The skin, too, can look sallow when our locks have lost their luster. The solution, of course, is to dye it, and by adding color to your hair, "you'll add color to your complexion," says Licari. But don't dive headfirst into the peroxide pool just yet; you'll first need to determine what kind of hair color commitment you're really willing to make. Ask yourself these questions before you open that box:

HOW HEALTHY IS MY HAIR RIGHT NOW?

If your hair is brittle, you may want to forgo a peroxide process—also known as permanent hair color—which opens (and further damages) the cuticle, the outermost layer of the hair shaft. Damaged hair is more prone to frizzies and flyaways and tends not to take color very well anyway. If you're concerned about your hair's condition, opt for a treatment that doesn't lift or strip your hair of its natural color (like a demi-permanent process) or one that conditions and adds shine, like a gloss or glaze. Fine hair, on the other hand, will get some added body from a color treatment.

WHAT IS MY HAIR'S TEXTURE?

This is particularly important for anyone looking to go lighter. Coarse, dark hair + peroxide does not equal platinum. "Asian women often wind up with orange hair after trying to go blond," says celebrity hair colorist Rona O'Connor, who has tinted the tresses of Brooke Shields and Christie Brinkley. Same goes for African American women—blond dye molecules don't easily penetrate the cuticles of thick, curly hair, resulting in a shade that looks more Orange Crush than baby blond. That doesn't mean you can't have sunny strands if you're a woman of color, however. Ask your colorist to paint the tips for a beachy effect. "A few highlights around the face is more flattering and easy to pull off, no matter what your ethnic background is," says O'Connor.

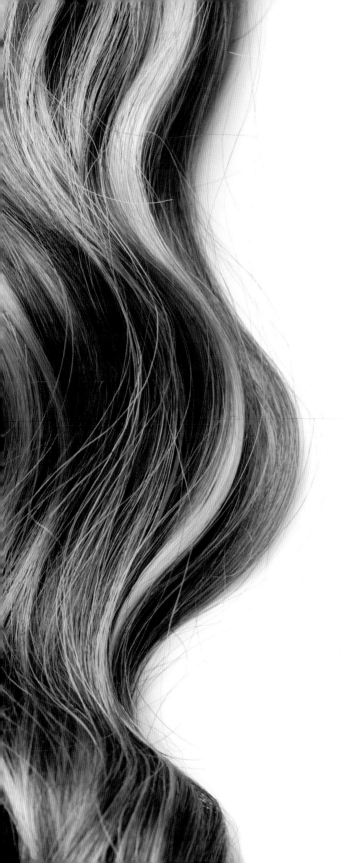

HOW WILL THE COLOR LOOK WITH ROOTS?

If getting to your colorist every three months is the most you can handle (or afford), be prepared to show your roots. Overgrown roots don't have to look trashy, however. In fact, they can even give your mane some depth and texture, depending on the shade of your base color. (Unfortunately, this doesn't work for me, since I have black hair.) At-home touch-ups can help you stretch the time between salon appointments, too.

AM I WILLING TO DO THE MAINTENANCE?

Some colors will require touch-ups every three to six weeks, and you'll need to be up for the task. Blond, for example, fades fast, while red can turn brassy. If you're not interested in developing a committed relationship with your colorist or devoting the time it takes to do it yourself, choose a process that's less high maintenance.

when blond actually ages you

Barbie-blond hair may be an okay look for the fifty-year-old plastic doll, but it's not a flattering shade on any woman north of thirty-five. "Women often get addicted to bleaching, and they want to go blonder and blonder," says Licari. "But platinum blond hair doesn't make you look younger. It has the opposite effect—it reads as white and it's instantly aging." (It's true! After moving to Los Angeles, I couldn't believe how often I'd notice a bleached blonde from behind, assume she was young, and then be shocked when she turned around to reveal an aging, sallow-skinned complexion. White blond is too severe a contrast next to older, paler skin.)

If you want to stay in the blond family, stick with a honey hue (rather than ash), and don't go beyond two shades lighter than your natural color. Still unsure which shade of blond is right for you? Consult a professional colorist—otherwise you may wind up in a salon seat anyway. Warns stylist Tippi Shorter, "Most of the people I see in the salon are in for color corrections."

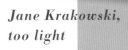

Jane Krakowski, too light

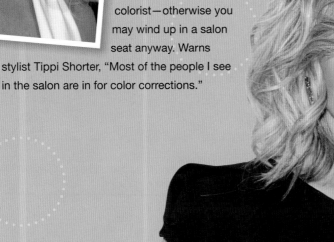

Just right

CHOOSING AN AT-HOME COLOR KIT

If You Want To...

* Go lighter
* Dramatically switch shades
* Cover hair that's more than 50 percent gray

Look For...

PERMANENT COLOR

These formulas typically contain ammonia and peroxide, chemicals that open the cuticle—the outermost layer of the hair strand—to deposit dye inside. As the name implies, permanent hair color is permanent; it will last until the hair grows out (or until you decide to chop it off), so you should take the plunge only if you're comfortable committing to a dramatic change and you're willing to have it touched up regularly.

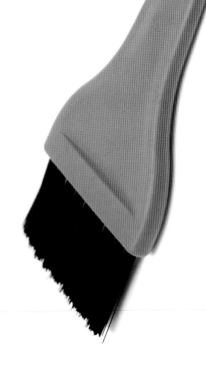

Try...

For salon effects: Frédéric Fekkai Salon Color, with its bowl and brush application, makes it easy to target roots and grays, while the herbal-infused formula contains an array of pigments, giving you rich, multidimensional color.

For quick results: Most permanent hair color takes twenty to thirty minutes, but L'Oréal Excellence to-Go takes just ten—even on stubborn gray hair—thanks to a low-ammonia technology that causes less breakage while sealing in color.

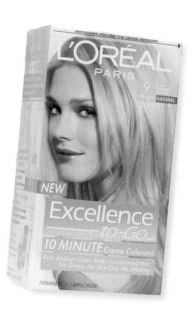

If You Want To...

⁕ Deepen, but not change existing color
⁕ Try a new hue without a full commitment
⁕ Cover hair that's between 20 and 50 percent gray

Look For...

DEMI-PERMANENT COLOR

Slightly gentler than a permanent formula, demi-permanent color contains little peroxide and no ammonia, so it coats the outside of the hair shaft with dye without lifting the natural color. These formulas typically wash out after twenty-eight shampoos.

Try...

Clairol's Natural Instincts contains antioxidants to soften hair while enhancing your natural color. The Brass Free line comes in six neutral to ashy shades that diminish orange and red tones without covering highlights.

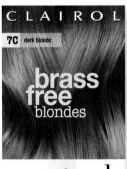

If You Want To...

⁕ Boost or brighten your own color with minimal upkeep
⁕ Cover hair that's less than 20 percent gray

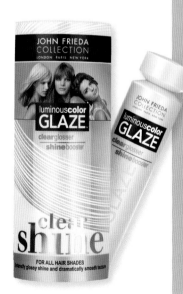

Look For...

GLAZE

Glazes are temporary tints that enhance your natural hair color by gently depositing mild dyes along the shaft. Light-reflecting ingredients also add shine.

Try...

John Frieda Collection Luminous Color Glaze comes in a variety of shades, so finding your color match is easy. Lather it on in the shower three times a week.

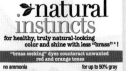

If You Want To...

* Add sun-kissed streaks
* Give flat color a little added dimension

Try...

Garnier Nutrisse Nourishing Multi-Lights offers four easy-to-wear shades that add subtle contrast while conditioning hair with avocado oil and vitamin E.

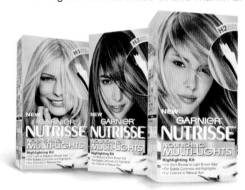

Look For...

HIGHLIGHTS

Highlights are created by strategically applying permanent color to small sections of the hair, great for creating a subtly lighter look or for adding depth and dimension.

do or dye: how to avoid common at-home color mistakes

Buy two boxes "You don't want to run out midway through an application," says colorist Sharon Dorram of Sally Hershberger Salon in New York City. "Buy more if your hair is long or thick."

Halve the time of your strand test Check the color way before the time is up. If you don't like it, wash it out immediately. If you do, let it sit for the full length of time.

Keep your skin safe While you're waiting for the dye to do its thing, tuck your hair back in a plastic shower cap and "pad the hairline with cotton so the dye doesn't leak beyond its perimeter," advises celebrity stylist David Evangelista, who represents Garnier Fructis. This is especially important if you have fair skin or if you're using a topical medication like Retin-A, which makes the skin more likely to "grab" color.

Touch up your roots while giving overall color a boost If you just need a root touch-up, target that area. With about five to ten minutes left to go before rinsing, apply color to the rest of the hair. "The older parts of your hair are more porous and will suck the dye in. You'll look uneven if you leave it on too long," says L'Oréal's Patty Slattery.

Don't try at-home color on a Friday night The help line may be closed for the weekend. Check the times on the box before using the product, advises Dorram.

How to Choose the Right Shade of At-Home Color

Whether you're contemplating a mane of a different color or you just want to cover some gray, selecting the right shade—from the hundreds of choices—can be more than a little intimidating. Cut through the clutter with these simple tips:

DO stay within two shades of your natural color It's the best way to make sure you're accenting your skin tone and eye color. Even if you're considering going from blond to brunette or vice versa, check the box and select a shade that's within your color family. You may need to lighten or deepen your color gradually, checking at each turn to make sure the shade still flatters your face.

DON'T match your hair color to your skin tone "Your hair color should be at least two shades darker than your natural skin tone," says Rona O'Connor. "Otherwise, you'll look washed out." If you find yourself compensating by piling on the makeup, it's time to deepen the shade.

DO a strand test Yes, it's a pain, but there's no more accurate way to determine if you've picked the right shade. Paint a few strands around your face so you can get a sense of how the shade interacts with your skin and eye color.

DON'T go too dark Unless you're naturally a rich brunette, going too dark can look too severe and add years to your age. Women who are fair-haired with a light complexion will be able to pull off a vampy look *only* if they have full lips, soft features, or blue, green, or hazel eyes, like Angelina Jolie or Jennifer Connelly. Women with slightly darker complexions should try a rich chocolate brown or caramel color.

DON'T try a major color overhaul at home Find a reputable colorist in your area and come armed with photos of women whose skin tone and eye color are similar to yours. Then ask for his or her honest opinion. "Sometimes our sense of what we look like isn't always reality," says Licari. "We all need the help of an impartial outsider."

DON'T worry about whether your skin tone is "warm" or "cool" "That old rule that a cool skin tone begets a cool hair shade isn't necessarily true," says O'Connor. "Blake Lively [of TV's *Gossip Girl*] has peaches-and-cream skin, but I gave her golden highlights to warm up her complexion." She also added warm tones to Daisy Fuentes's brunette mane, to downplay the cool, greenish cast of her olive skin. When in doubt, mix warm and cool tones.

DO consider going red Just as blush can perk up the face, some auburn or strawberry highlights—especially on women with ivory skin—can turn up the volume on blah hair color and wake up your complexion. "This works best on women who have pink undertones to their skin; it will play up the pink and add blush to the cheeks," says O'Connor.

Black Hair: Basic Care and Styling

Because the natural oils produced by the scalp don't move as easily down the shaft of kinky, curly, or textured strands, African American women may struggle with hair that's dry, fragile, and increasingly prone to breakage. Top stylists Ursula Stephen (who has worked with stars like Rihanna, Mary J. Blige, Monica, and Paula Patton) and Tippi Shorter (Alicia Keys, Jennifer Hudson) share their secrets to maintaining a healthy, stylish mane.

BASIC CARE

To avoid stripping the hair of its natural moisture, Stephen recommends shampooing no more than once a week. Before you start, soak the hair thoroughly in very hot water to break up any excess oil. Then reach for a volumizing shampoo (try Rene Furterer Volumea shampoo to create body and fullness) and lather in a dime-sized amount from the nape to the crown. Repeat. "The first time is for the scalp," says Stephen. "The second time is for the hair." Rinse thoroughly.

Next, work in a dollop of conditioner, starting at the ends and moving to midshaft, using a wide-tooth comb to gently detangle until the hair feels smooth and soft. Rinse well and then ring out the hair in the shower. Towel-dry, blotting out any excess moisture, and spritz in a volumizing spray.

Once a month, switch to a clarifying shampoo to remove any product residue.

STYLING PREP

Since you're shampooing only once a week, you'll need a bit of a refresher before styling your hair for an evening out. To dissolve excess product and remove any oil, spray on a little Ojon Dry Recovery Revitalizing Moisture Mist, aiming at the roots (for chemically straightened hair, try TRESemmé Fresh Start Dry Shampoo). Then rake your fingers through your hair and "power dry," the preferred method of Shorter: Dip your head over, tousle the hair from roots to ends, and move a blow-dryer all around your head. If you're going for a straight style, use a paddle brush instead of your fingers. Then choose your style:

For Bouncy Waves

Even if your hair is superthick, you can still get lustrous, loose waves without much fuss. The trick? Start by dividing the hair into six big sections. If you have dry hair, add a pea-sized amount of serum into each section—Biosilk Silk Therapy Serum is a good one—working it up from the ends to midshaft. If you have fine hair, try a light-hold spray, aiming it at the roots and brushing through to the ends (this will keep your hair from feeling crunchy). Or for added gloss, try a shine spray, like Ojon Shine & Protect Glossing Mist.

EASY CUT #1: THE PIXIE

Take a page out of Halle Berry's playbook and try this flattering, fast-styling cut. For curly hair, opt for a close-cropped style (think Beyoncé's little sis, Solange Knowles).

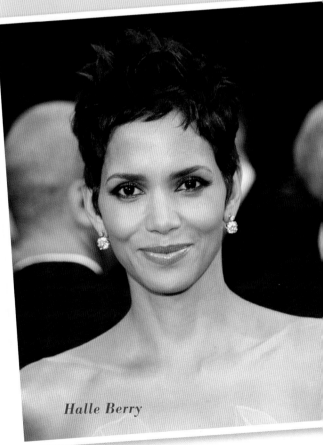

Halle Berry

EASY CUT #2: THE LONG BOB

Shorter recommends a layered, choppy bob to avoid the dreaded pyramid effect. If your hair is straightened or relaxed, a side-swept bang can help soften the face. Avoid bangs if your hair is curly, however; you'll wind up looking like you stepped off the set of *Flashdance*.

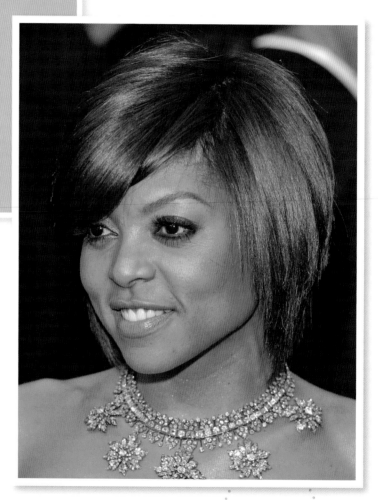

Taraji P. Henson

Next, wrap the sections in jumbo hot rollers (try the large rollers from BaByliss PRO and secure with butterfly clamps) and allow to set for fifteen minutes. Remove rollers and soften the curl with a paddle brush or, for more wave, a round natural-bristle brush.

For Sleek and Straight

For a stick-straight mane, start by spraying a dry shampoo at the roots, massaging it in with your fingers—this will dissolve oil on the scalp, so you won't be stuck fighting curls and waves caused by that excess moisture. Then apply an anti-frizz serum (like Pantene Anti-Frizz Straightening Crème) to add shine and protect the hair from heat styling. Emulsify a dollop in your hands and run it down the shaft of the hair, avoiding the roots. Use a paddle brush to get the strands as flat and straight as possible.

Next, reach for your flat iron—divide the hair into eight to ten sections and, with the temperature set at 250 degrees, try for a single pass through the hair. If you find yourself having to iron the same strands over and over, increase the heat in increments of 50 degrees, but don't allow the iron to sit on any spot for longer than five seconds. "It's like ironing your clothes," says Shorter. "You have to keep it moving, or you'll fry the hair."

If your hair is naturally curly and you're concerned about frizz (especially if you're expecting a rain shower), run a bit of the anti-frizz serum through the hair once more. Or, if your hair is very thick, you can set with a lightweight hair spray.

BEDTIME PREP

Before you hit the hay, brush your hair into a beehive-like bun and secure with a silk or cotton scarf. "I recommend silk because it retains moisture, but if you wash your hair less frequently, it might tend to get oily and go limp," says Stephen. If that's the case, use a cotton scarf in between shampoos to absorb any grease.

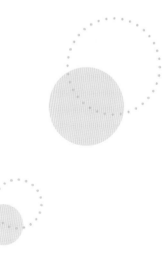

EASY CUT #3:
THE LIBERTY

Long layers work well for both natural waves and relaxed hair. A blunt-cut fringe (like Jennifer Hudson's) can draw attention to the eyes, while a side-swept bang is best for round, heart-, or square-shaped faces.

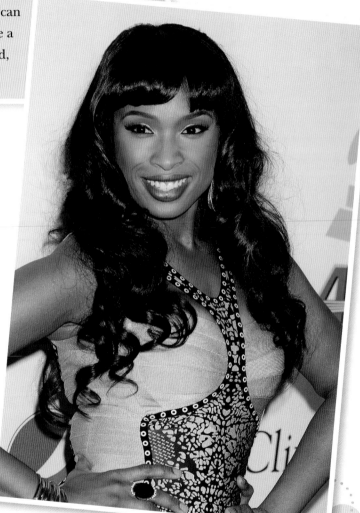

Jennifer Hudson

the 6 top hair essentials

Celebrity stylist Dominick Pucciarello identifies the top styling tools every mom needs to have on hand to stay well-tressed.

Shampoos and Conditioners

The best deals around—according to Pucciarello—are the products from Pantene. "The ingredients are good, and they leave the hair feeling soft and shiny."

Dry Shampoo

Though most hairdressers consider dry shampoo an essential tool for reviving dirty, oily hair on off-days, Pucciarello also uses Oribe's Apres Beach Spray to give his clients sexy, beachy waves. "It's my go-to product right now," he says. "It soaks up oil without looking waxy. You can spray it on and allow the hair to air dry, or apply it after blow-drying to get a polished wave."

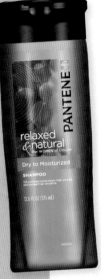

Brush

A round or flat boar bristle brush is key, since boar bristles polish the hair while providing enough tension during blow-drying to prevent flyaways and frizz. Pucciarello likes Ibiza brand brushes (available at amazon.com).

Mousse

"Paul Mitchell Foaming Mousse is still one of my favorites," says Pucciarello. "It smells great, adds just enough body for limp hair, and keeps curls from frizzing. Plus, you can find it in your local drugstore."

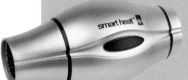

Hair Spray

Choose one labeled light-hold or "dry," and you'll still be able to run your fingers through your hair.

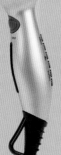

Blow-dryer

"Essential!" says Pucciarello. He recommends ionic dryers, which emit negatively charged ions and help the cuticle lie flat. Using the nozzle attachment—that piece you usually throw away or lose!—is also key: "This blows the air in one direction, keeping the cuticle of your hair in one direction, too, not blowing all over the place."

From Drab to Fab! Hot Mom Makeovers

These busy mothers may be short on time, but thanks to a trio of top-notch experts—celebrity hairstylist Ted Gibson, who tends to such A-listers as Anne Hathaway, Renée Zellweger, and Angelina Jolie; colorist Jason Backe; and makeup artist Brian Duprey—they're no longer short on style.

My husband sent a photo to his family that day, saying I looked great.

LISA

The Challenge "I often skimp on drying my hair and end up with a frizzy mess," said mom of two Lisa Broock, a magazine editor. "I wanted a low-maintenance, chic back-to-work style and color that won't wash me out."

The Cut A sassy, long-layered bob with bangs.

The Color Strawberry blond with highlights to bring out a rosy glow.

The Makeup Taupe shadow and nude gloss.

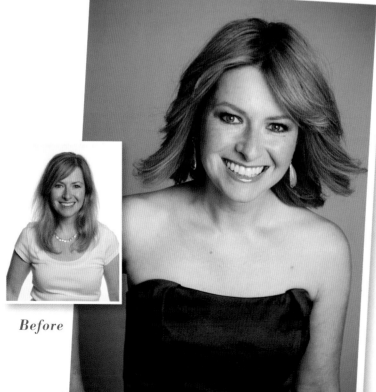

Before

After

ANNA

The Challenge "I'm a no-fuss, wash-and-go girl," said graphic designer (and mom to toddler Jagger James) Anna Valencia-Bruch. "I haven't had a serious haircut since I became a mom. I have no time to primp at home."

The Cut Gibson chopped off seven inches. "It will look great even in a ponytail because the layers are long and face framing," he says.

The Color Backe amped up shine with a blue black color treatment.

The Makeup Gunmetal gel liner on upper and lower lashes and a blackberry stain on the lips.

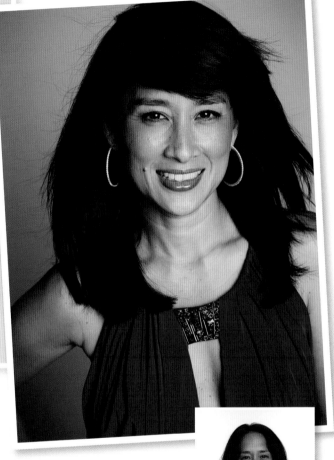

After

Before

> My son gave me a ton of kisses—I'll take that as a thumbs-up. And my husband loved it!

SUSAN

The Challenge Susan Petrie-Badertscher, founder of Petrie Point Designs (petriepointdesigns.com) and mom of two to daughter Lily and son Beckett, said she wanted to look less "hippie chick" and more "blond bombshell."

The Cut A modern layered 'do with wispy, angled side bangs. "It still looks good even when you're in a hurry," says Gibson. "Work in a little styling lotion, then air-dry."

The Color A honey base with golden highlights. "It instantly brightened up her face," says Backe.

The Makeup Gold shadow and a sheer apricot gloss.

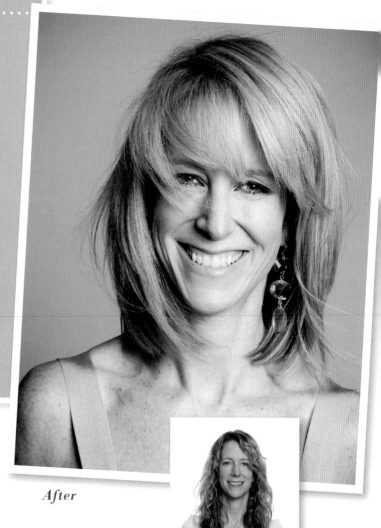

After

Before

JENNIFER

The Challenge Just six weeks after giving birth to daughter Kiera, education consultant Jennifer Grolemund was diagnosed with thyroid cancer. "I'm fine now, but the medicine made my hair thin," she said.

The Cut A low-maintenance graduated bob with side-swept bangs. "Blow-drying my hair forward from the back gives it body," she said.

The Color A hazelnut base enhanced by dark, medium, and light blond highlights.

The Makeup Shimmery nude smoky eyes and a raspberry high-shine lip balm.

My husband has no poker face, so when I saw his big smile, I knew he loved it!

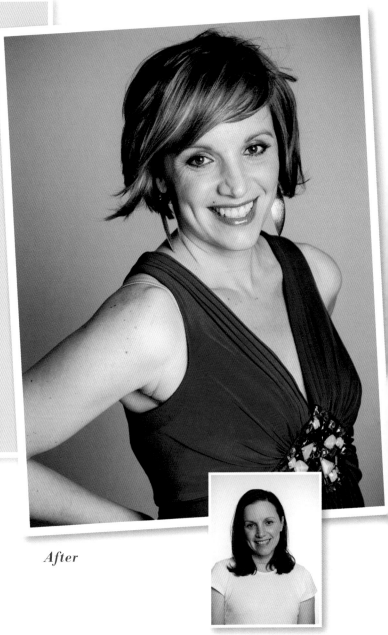

After

Before

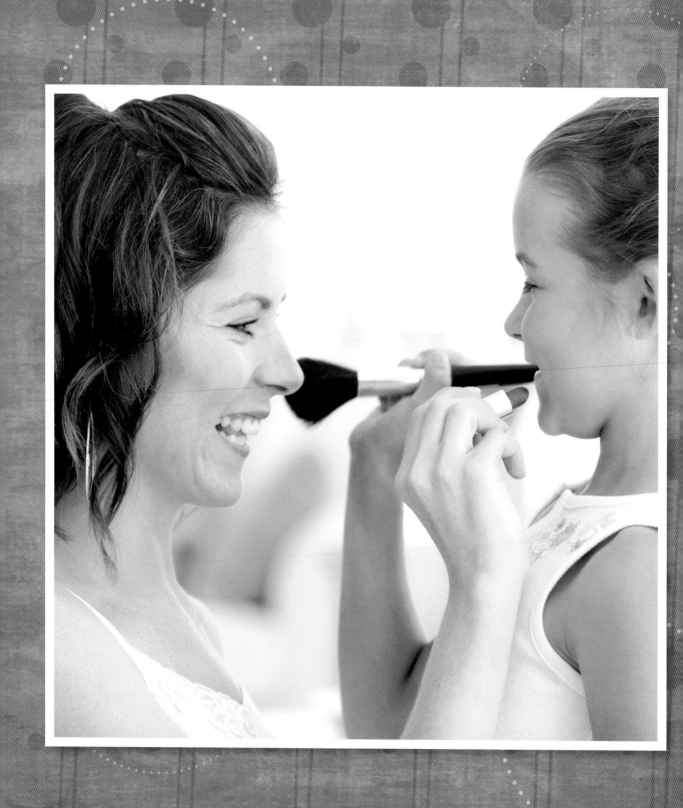

hot mess? try the 5-minute mom face

Fake a Good Night's Sleep with Easy Makeup

One of the perks of my job is to have my makeup professionally done before events and TV appearances. A makeup artist will arrive with a stash of products so large that it often requires a suitcase with wheels. And then for a full hour or so you get daubed and dabbed with every kind of tool imaginable: Not one, but two or maybe even three colors of foundation are mixed before it dare touch your skin. Later, a Michelangelo-at-the-Sistine-Chapel scenario goes on with your eyelids; the shadow application alone can take upward of twenty minutes. Even though the experience can be fun, it also can be deeply humbling. One of the makeup artists I really like in L.A. always starts by applying dark contour all around the perimeter of my face to "make it look smaller." (I can only assume she thinks my face is fat.) Others will discuss their techniques out loud, saying things like "This will hide those dark circles" when I had no idea my eyes looked tired. Minor humiliation notwithstanding, the end result is that I look like a much, much better version of myself after one of these sessions—like someone with perfect skin, beautiful, thick lashes, and no trace of that big zit I woke up with.

Every time I get my makeup done, I'm reminded a bit of what it was like to be a young girl, back when I first started experimenting with cosmetics. In the pre-text-message age (when every tween seemed to have much more free time), I would spend hours lovingly and painstakingly organizing my Bonne Bell cola-flavored lip glosses or wet n wild eye shadows and trying on different looks all night long in front of the mirror. I knew the names of every color of lipstick I had (not to mention the brand name, as well as where I bought it), and—despite not being much of a girly-girl—I still loved poring over the cosmetics at the grocery or drugstore while my mom was busy shopping.

Now, of course, my relationship with makeup has changed completely. The makeup drawer in my bathroom (which is so messy it looks like a burglary has occurred) is packed with broken items, ugly colors, forgotten lipsticks (it's tragic how often I find items I somehow forgot about or, worse, bought twice), and eye shadow

brushes that I am quite certain have not been washed in the recommended time frame. Or ever. And in the morning, no matter what day of the week, I am always rushing to beat the clock, in a near panic just to get myself presentable before I have to walk out the door. Sometimes I have fifteen minutes. Sometimes I have just five. If anyone told me when I was twenty-two that one day I would have to get two children fed, dressed, and out the door by eight A.M., I would have laughed at them and hit the snooze button.

So, knowing the time constraints from which we all suffer, as well as the almost universal desire to look "naturally" pretty (instead of wildly overdone), I devote this chapter to revealing what the experts know (and we don't) about looking your best in the least amount of time. "Makeup should never steal the show," says celebrity makeup artist Fiona Stiles, who has worked with Elizabeth Banks, Nikki Reed, and Gabrielle Union. "When you think of someone like Halle Berry, she always looks effortlessly pulled together, which makes you think she has it all under control." In the end, you might even fool people into thinking you had all the time in the world.

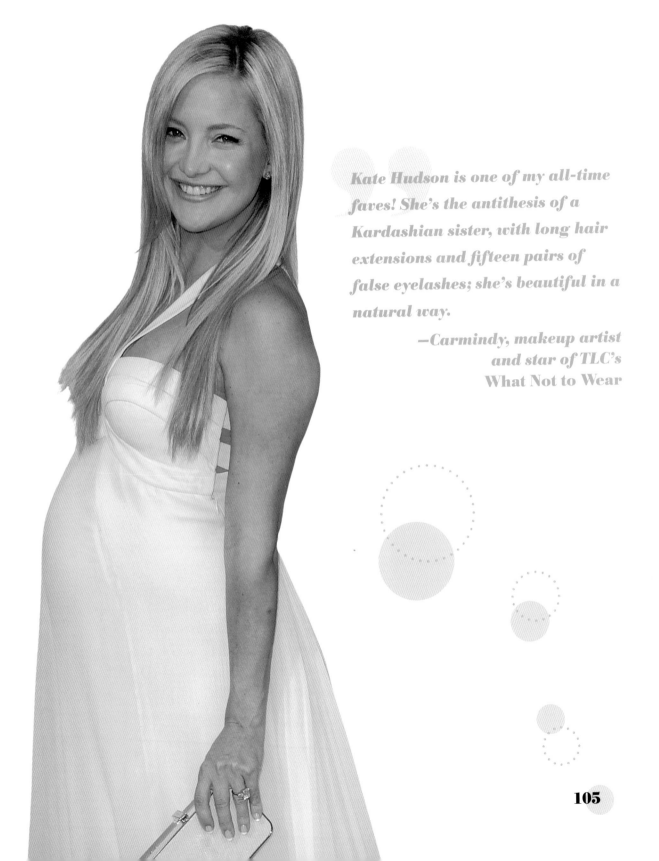

Kate Hudson is one of my all-time faves! She's the antithesis of a Kardashian sister, with long hair extensions and fifteen pairs of false eyelashes; she's beautiful in a natural way.

—Carmindy, makeup artist
and star of TLC's
What Not to Wear

105

You: From Hot Mess to Hot Mom...in 5 Minutes Flat

Erasing the signs of sleep deprivation and evening out your complexion shouldn't take more than mere moments, according to celebrity makeup artist Carmindy, author of *The 5-Minute Face* and star of TLC's *What Not to Wear*. Start by cleansing and applying a moisturizer with SPF. Then follow these steps for a flawless morning face, fast!

STEP 1
PRIME YOUR CANVAS

Begin by applying a light layer of liquid foundation, using a latex sponge to blend in evenly and smooth out the skin tone. Then reach for a cream highlighting pen. What's that, you ask? Highlighters are sheer and shimmery, and by depositing light-diffusing particles on the face, they can even out and brighten the skin, draw attention to the eyes, and help you look more rested. "It's the key to enhancing natural beauty," says Carmindy. Choose one in a shade slightly lighter than your natural skin tone. If you're fair, opt for a pink or champagne color. For those with olive or darker complexions, try gold. Then tap it in three places: under the eyebrow, inside the corner of the eye, and right on top of the cheekbone.

My favorite highlighting pens are the admittedly pricey Yves Saint Laurent Touche Éclat and LORAC Double Feature (concealer on one end, highlighter on the other), but you can get similar results (without breaking the bank) with Revlon's Age Defying Spa Concealer.

STEP 2
FAKE A NATURAL FLUSH

Cream blushes work best on most skin because they don't get stuck in the pores (the way some gels can) or cake (the way some powders do). Since a little goes a long way, just dip your index finger in the pot and tap on the fleshy apple of your cheeks. Opt for peachy shades, which flatter pale to dark complexions and tend to look more natural in the daylight. (Try Maybelline Dream Mousse Blush in Peach Satin.)

STEP 3
ACCENT YOUR EYES

If you're just out running errands or shuttling the kids from school to swim lessons, you really don't need the coverage (or even the color) of eye shadow—a quick pump of an eyelash curler (a tool Carmindy calls "a must") and a swipe of black mascara (on the upper lashes only) is enough for daytime. If you have dark lids, visible veins or blood vessels, or if the skin of your eyelid is crepey, a few dabs of an eye shadow primer can even out the skin tone and give you a more polished look. Try Laura Mercier Eye Basics in Wheat for a near-universal shade.

STEP 4
GROOM YOUR BROWS

Take a moment to fill in any bare spots in the brow with a few light strokes of an eyebrow pencil (choose a shade slightly lighter than your actual brow color so you don't wind up looking like Herman Munster), then shape your arches with a clear brow gel (these typically look like a clear mascara), which will keep them in place throughout the day. "Busy women are sometimes tempted to skip this step," says Stiles, "but if your brows look polished, so will you. And it takes all of two seconds."

STEP 5
PLAY UP YOUR POUT

The secret to kissable lips is to look dewy, not done. On "school days," all you really need is a swipe of rose-hued gloss or tinted balm (I like Tarte 24.7 Natural Lip Sheer, available at Sephora and tartecosmetics.com). For a pucker with slightly more impact, try a sheer or slightly pearlescent red or berry shade of lipstick. Just be sure to avoid matte pinks and harsh corals, which don't flatter sallow skin. And steer clear of frosted lipsticks—they're both dated and aging.

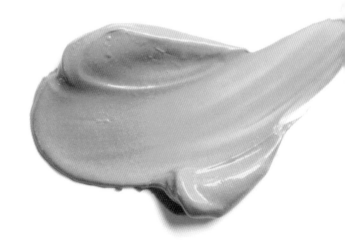

Old Mom Vs. Modern Mom

Remember all those women who played the mom in movies and TV shows from the 1950s and 1960s, who looked as if their entire face had been painted on with a thick-bristled brush? Women who, if they fell asleep with their makeup still on, would probably wake up with a perfect image of their face imprinted on their pillowcase? These days, nothing will age you more than wearing too much makeup (or the wrong *kinds* of makeup). Don't get caught making these common mom mistakes!

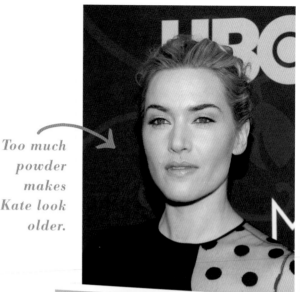

Too much powder makes Kate look older.

OLD MOM

Powder foundation for a flat, no-glow complexion

MODERN MOM

Youthful, dewy skin

While a light dusting of translucent powder can help *set* your makeup, heavy powder foundations are out—they tend to cake and settle in fine lines and wrinkles (making them more noticeable), and the matte look instantly makes you look older. (A natural, dewy glow, after all, is a sign of youth.) Whether it comes in an airbrush spray or a bottle, liquid foundation is better.

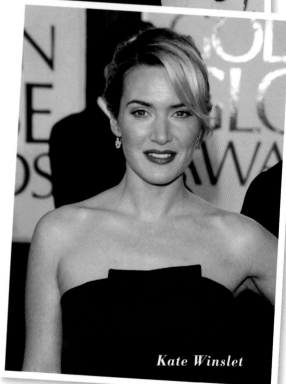

Kate Winslet

OLD MOM
All-over bronzer

MODERN MOM
A subtle, sun-kissed glow

Women who love to cover their faces in clay-colored bronzer may *think* they're replicating a tropical glow, but too much makeup just makes the skin appear dull, dirty, and old. (I always think about the neighbor in *There's Something About Mary*.) If you'd like to look sun-kissed, there's a strategic way to apply bronzer: Use a wide-bristle brush to dust it on in a "C" shape, starting at the temples, sweeping down along the hairline, and ending right under the cheekbone. "Moderation is the key," says Carmindy.

Too much bronzer!

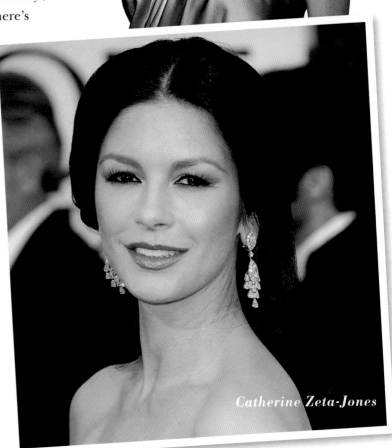

Catherine Zeta-Jones

OLD MOM
Overplucked, barely-there brows

MODERN MOM
Well-groomed arches

Scant, sparse, barely-there brows will make you look ancient, or worse, just plain weird. Even so—according to Carmindy—"there's an epidemic of overplucked brows in this country." A full brow, however, provides your face with a frame and takes years off your age. To avoid overplucking, try using your tweezers no more than once a week, and tweeze stray hairs only below the natural arch.

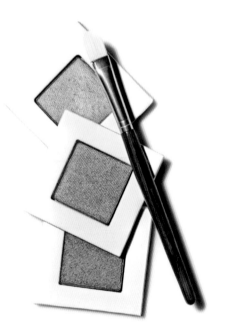

OLD MOM
Frosted or pastel-hued eye shadow

MODERN MOM
Neutral shades with shimmer

With the thousands of shades, textures, and formulas available, you may be tempted to purchase eye shadow in an array of candy-colored hues. Resist this urge, says Carmindy. "Easter egg shades look unnatural and old-fashioned, and pink shadow makes you look bloodshot and tired."

When you *do* want to add a little more drama to the eye, try a shimmer—rather than a frosted—shadow in neutral shades like gray, taupe, or brown. How to tell the difference? Put some of the product on the back of your hand. "If you see confetti squares," says Carmindy, "then it's frosted, and it'll look too severe. If you see a liquidy luminescence, that's a shimmer; it's a more finely milled powder and it'll create a softer, more youthful glow."

OLD MOM
Dark, heavy eyeliner on the lower lash line

MODERN MOM
Eyes lined with a neutral taupe

This rocker chick makeup staple *should* have gone the way of your stonewashed jeans and ripped concert T-shirts—rimming the inside of your lower lash line makes the eye appear smaller and emphasizes dark undereye circles. (Dark brown or black liners tend to look too harsh on older women or women with very fair complexions anyway.) To create the illusion of big, bright eyes without looking like Marilyn Manson's mother, try using a neutral taupe, like Mineral Fusion Touch Eye Pencil (available at Whole Foods), which will still add dimension and depth even when used on darker skin tones. "It's my secret weapon," says Fiona Stiles of the barely-there shade. "Plus, you don't have to worry about drawing a perfectly precise line when using a lighter color." For a slightly more dramatic look, use an angle brush to smudge on a chocolate brown shadow, but *only* along the upper lash line. "Then quickly swipe your finger across the line," says Carmindy. "You'll be left with just a hint of color and the illusion of a thicker lash line."

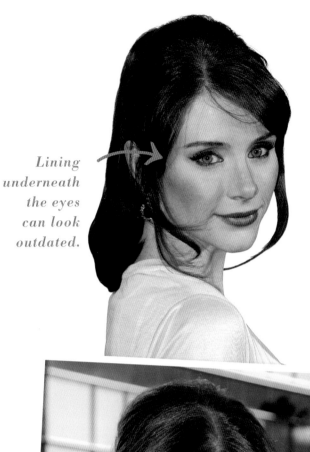

Lining underneath the eyes can look outdated.

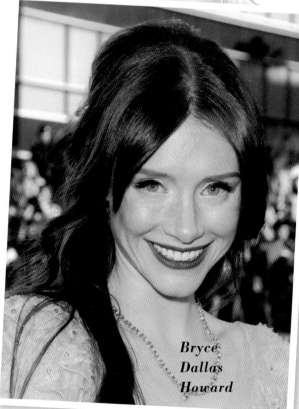

Bryce Dallas Howard

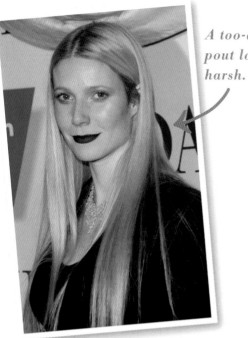

A too-dark pout looks harsh.

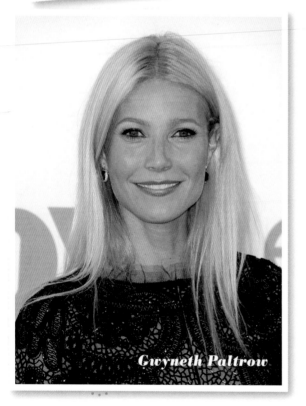

Gwyneth Paltrow

OLD MOM
A harsh, opaque pout

MODERN MOM
Kissable lips

If, as a little girl, you ever watched in wonder as your mother carefully applied her lipstick, it probably went something like this: Rim the entire lip and then fill in with a harsh liner pencil. Swipe on two coats of a thick, goopy stick. Blot with a tissue, then smile at the mirror and check for signs of color on the teeth. Well, mothers don't always know best—a supermatte mouth can make your lips look small, dry, and downright clownlike (and the darker the color, the more likely it is to feather and bleed). For a kissable mouth, swap your opaque lipsticks for sheer, shimmery glosses in berry tones. You'll look so much younger. Promise!

mom skin SOS

For an Angry Pimple

Whatever you do, don't pop it! You've heard it umpteen times before—and it's *still* hard to resist—but picking at your pimples can lead to scarring and infection. Instead, use a concealer brush (rather than your fingers) to apply a drying concealer, which will stay put longer than a creamy formula. Try Laura Mercier's Secret Camouflage. For nighttime treatment, I like Clinique Acne Solutions Spot Healing Gel.

For Puffy Eyes

Up crying late last night? Or maybe that was just the baby. Either way, swollen lids are telltale signs of sleep deprivation, but who has the time to lie on her back with a couple of cucumbers balanced on her eyeballs? Instead, soak a few teabags in hot water (chamomile acts as an anti-inflammatory) and store them in the fridge. Next time you're feeling a bit puffy, take one out and hold it against your eyelids for a minute or so to draw down the swelling. (Fresh out of tea? Keep a spoon or two in the freezer—they'll work in a pinch too.)

If you're still feeling a little puffy, avoid light shades of eye shadow as well as anything that shimmers; the shine will only draw attention to the swelling. Instead, blend a chocolate brown or black liner right at the lashes and sweep on a coat of mascara. "Thick lashes can help camouflage puffy skin," says Stiles. "Mascara is a terrific diversion."

For Oily Skin

Not every woman in the world needs a moisturizer in the morning, so if your makeup usually slides off your face by eleven A.M., skip it. "Your oil glands are already producing your own moisturizer anyway," says Stiles. Same goes for "luminizing" foundations you might find at the drugstore—all of your cosmetics should be labeled "oil-free." And instead of taming that shine with regular pressed powder, try blotting papers—like Neutrogena Shine-Control Blotting Sheets, which won't disturb your makeup—or MAC Blot Powder compact, which won't cake on top of your foundation. "I give these to all my clients for the red carpet," says Stiles. The only thing not to skip is sunscreen. Neutrogena Dry-Touch Sunblocks are great for avoiding a greasy face.

For Skin That Looks Sallow

Whether you're sleep- or sun-deprived, you don't have to advertise it. A bit of blush or bronzer is the easiest way to wake up a tired face. Dot your cheekbones with a cream blush, or sweep a powder blush across the apples of your cheeks. "A little gradual self-tanner will also knock out that greenish cast in a day or two," adds Stiles. Try St. Tropez Everyday Gradual Tan Face.

What Happens to Your Skin...

Lots of women have preconceived notions of what it's like to be pregnant; one of the most pervasive is the idea that expectant mothers spend nine months floating around in some kind of angelic, ethereal cloud—we've all heard of the "pregnancy glow," and we've all been led to believe that we should be at our most beautiful when we're with child. (That "glow," by the way, *does* have a medical basis: During pregnancy, your body is busy circulating 50 percent more blood than usual, and all that extra blood carries extra oxygen to the surface of your skin. Basically, getting pregnant is like getting the best oxygen facial of your life.) Fluctuating hormones, however, can cause a range of annoying skin afflictions—from acne to stretch marks to skin tags—both during and after pregnancy. In fact, your skin may freak out even *before* you conceive, since coming off the pill has been known to trigger a breakout of blemishes.

Acne

The most common pregnancy-related skin ailment—without question—is acne. Most oral acne treatments, however, as well as topical ingredients—including salicylic acid (more than 2 percent), retinoid creams (like Retin-A), and antibiotics—are out, at least until after you've finished breastfeeding. So what's left on the menu?

Though you should always speak with your doctor before trying any new product while pregnant or breastfeeding, topical glycolic acid is generally considered safe to use, as is benzoyl peroxide in low concentrations. For stubborn breakouts, some doctors also may prescribe a topical erythromycin cream, which *is* an antibiotic but is also considered safe. An ounce of prevention goes a long way, too. Clean your face twice a day with a gentle, nonmedicated cleanser, and make sure all of your cosmetics, especially foundation, are labeled oil-free and noncomedogenic (meaning not known to cause acne). If you weren't prone to breakouts before getting pregnant, then your baby-related acne should subside somewhere around seven months after delivery, when your hormone levels have returned to normal.

Stretch Marks

Though there's not much evidence to suggest that stretch marks can be *prevented* (even by cocoa butter creams and other "miracle" products), one way you can help lessen the likelihood of developing these pink, raised, and often itchy scars is to try to pace your pregnancy weight gain. Stretch marks form when the skin is stretched too fast, causing the elastic fibers to snap; you'll be more likely to develop them if you gain weight in fits and starts rather than slow and steady.

Stretch marks, which occur in up to 90 percent of pregnant women, will gradually lighten and fade on their own, but to speed up that process, try Mederma Stretch Marks Therapy. Once you've finished breastfeeding, prescription-strength Retin-A also can help lighten the unsightly lines.

Skin Tags

Skin tags, those floppy little pieces of skin that often show up on the neck, under the breasts, between your thighs, or under your armpits, may be unsightly, but they're totally harmless. Even though you can't prevent them—skin tags are triggered by friction, like skin rubbing against skin, as well as by hormone fluctuations, which is why they're common during pregnancy—and you can't

really treat them (no home surgery—don't try to get rid of them yourself!), they can be easily and painlessly removed by a dermatologist.

Spider Veins

As we discussed in chapter 1, changes in circulation, as well as an increase in the amount of blood pumping through your body, can cause clusters of red- or blue-tinted spider veins to spring up on your legs, hips, and thighs. While laser treatments can minimize or eliminate the veins (but only after you've delivered), a spray-on bronzer or leg makeup like Sally Hansen Airbrush Legs can make them less noticeable—and it's certainly less costly.

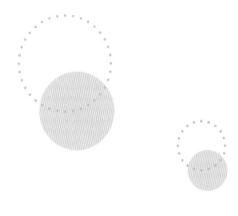

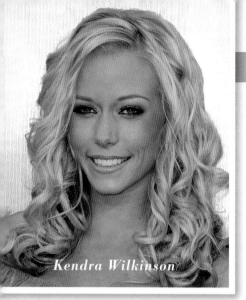

Kendra Wilkinson

Women in their twenties tend to have a complexion that's naturally radiant; so at this age, your skin care routine should focus more on *prevention* than treatment. To stave off future sun damage, and fine lines and wrinkles, make the daily application of sunscreen your number-one priority. "It's worth thousands in the antiaging bank," says Ellen Marmur, M.D., chief of dermatologic and cosmetic surgery at Mount Sinai Medical Center in New York. Sun protection becomes doubly important if you use a topical antibiotic for acne (since these may make your skin more sensitive to the sun), if you're on birth control pills, or if you're planning to become pregnant—melasma, which causes stubborn brown spots and unsightly dark patches on the face, is triggered by fluctuating hormones (including synthetic hormones in the pill) in combination with sun exposure.

Forget about choosing a high SPF, however, and reach for a broad-spectrum block with ingredients like zinc or titanium dioxide; these will protect your skin from both UVA *and* UVB rays. "People get a false sense of protection by using a higher SPF," says dermatologist Neal Schultz, M.D. "But there's really no need to go beyond SPF 15, which provides 88 percent protection against burning rays. The most important thing is to reapply every three to four hours or after swimming, since no sunscreen is *really* waterproof."

The most common skin complaints of women in their twenties are oily skin, large pores, and acne blemishes. If you struggle with blackheads, choose a cleanser with salicylic acid, an anti-inflammatory that will help reduce redness. If you tend to develop whiteheads, try one with benzoyl peroxide. Hormonal acne, on the other hand, which typically appears on the chin and jawline, can be resistant to creams and gels. If you often experience breakouts timed with your menstrual period, talk to your doctor about switching birth control. Some forms of the pill have been approved to treat acne.

A ruddy or blemish-prone complexion also may benefit from regular exercise. "All that sweating flushes everything out and helps unclog the pores," says Dr. Marmur. "Exercise also improves circulation, regulates your mood, decreases stress, and helps you sleep better—all things that affect the look and feel of the skin."

As you enter your thirties, the skin's natural process of exfoliation starts to slow down, which is why fine lines and wrinkles may become more pronounced and any sun damage you accumulated in your teens and twenties will start to show. "The keyword now is 'multitask,' " says Dr. Marmur. Upgrade your regular moisturizer/SPF combo to one that *also* includes antiaging ingredients; topical antioxidants, for example, can enhance SPF protection and inhibit free radical damage during the day, as well as help repair sun damage at night. (Try Aveeno Positively Ageless Youth Perfecting Moisturizer with SPF 30 or Garnier Nutritioniste Skin Renew Anti-Sun-Damage Daily Moisture Lotion with SPF 28.) To further fight blotchiness, brown spots, and uneven skin tone, slough away any lingering dead skin cells with a creamy exfoliator—St. Ives Apricot Scrub is a good one—but no more than once or twice a week. (Chemical scrubs, which utilize harsher ingredients like alpha hydroxy acid, may irritate sensitive skin.)

Something else to keep in mind: It's not uncommon for women in their thirties to suddenly develop skin allergies and irritations, particularly when they're pregnant. In fact, Dr. Marmur estimates that between shampoo, perfume, makeup, and skin care products, our skin gets exposed

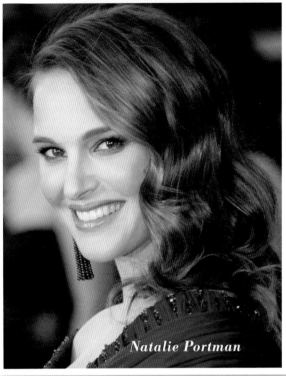

Natalie Portman

to upward of 120 different chemicals a day. If you're experiencing rashes or other breakouts, consider giving your skin a cosmetic detox—a two- or three-day break from your regular products—and then getting back to what's really essential. "We tend to apply more and more antiaging products as we enter this age bracket," says Dr. Marmur. "But less is really more."

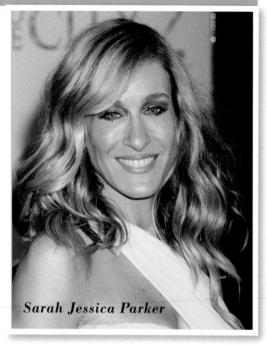

Sarah Jessica Parker

By the time we hit forty, our natural skin cell turnover—the rate at which old cells slough off and new cells emerge—has slowed significantly, from somewhere around twenty-eight days (when you're still in your thirties) to more like forty days. Since those dead cells are hanging around on your face for a longer period of time, your complexion may begin to dull, and lines and wrinkles can become increasingly pronounced. In other words, "this is the age when skin care starts to get serious," says Dr. Marmur. Products that are designed to boost your skin's surface cell turnover rate, like the Olay Professional Pro-X line, can help you get your glow back.

Dry skin also becomes a growing concern for woman in their forties and beyond, especially as you move into perimenopause—plummeting estrogen contributes to dry skin, as well as hot flashes and flushing, thinning skin, and more visible pores. If you're looking to remove makeup, banish bar soaps (they tend to be drying) in favor of a moisturizing cleansing milk, like Clinique's Take the Day Off Cleansing Milk, or alcohol-free baby wipes. If your skin is flaky, try soaking a nubby washcloth in warm water and then lathering with a moisturizing lotion. "Massage it gently onto the face," says Dr. Marmur. "This will exfoliate and hydrate the skin, as well as help drain the lymphatic system to de-puff the delicate undereye area."

To fight dark patches and blotchy pigmentation, retinoid creams (like Retin-A and Renova) are some of the most effective products on the market; bear in mind, however, that retinoid creams cannot be used while you are pregnant. Since these creams may irritate sensitive skin, it's best to start off slow with a mild, nonprescription formula.

The 20 Best Everyday Products

Let's say you needed to make a last-minute batch of cupcakes for your child's classroom party... *tomorrow.* Alas, you don't have all the ingredients. Think how much time and energy you'll waste running around trying to find the perfect-colored frosting and just the right sprinkles. The same principle applies when you're trying to simplify the process of getting ready in the morning. Step one? Making sure you have the very best tools at your fingertips.

CERAVE HYDRATING CLEANSER

"When it comes to washing your face, you actually don't want squeaky clean," insists New York dermatologist Dr. David Colbert. He recommends this gentle, noncomedogenic cleanser, which will cut through makeup and wipe away grime, excess oil, and dead skin cells, all without upsetting your natural moisture balance or irritating dry or acne-prone skin. Plus, it feels as creamy and elegant as a pricey spa brand. Available at drugstores nationwide.

LA ROCHE-POSAY ANTHELIOS SX SPF 15 DAILY MOISTURIZING CREAM WITH SUNSCREEN

This European sunblock was once so coveted in the States, beauty insiders would hoard it in their suitcases after trips abroad. These days you can find it at any CVS—and it affords unparalleled protection against UVA *and* UVB rays, thanks to an organic filter called Mexoryl SX. This magical stuff doesn't degrade as quickly as some other sunscreens, which means you'll have a higher protection factor for a longer period of time. "You don't need an SPF higher than 15," assures Dr. Colbert. The formula also blends in seamlessly, without leaving a white film on your skin.

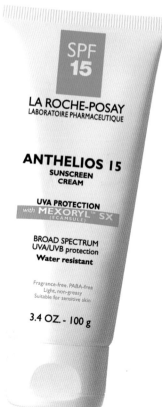

DR. HAUSCHKA DAILY REVITALIZING EYE CREAM

When choosing an eye cream, you'll want to steer clear of formulas that come loaded with too many perks, like alpha hydroxy acid, which can irritate the sensitive eye area. This soothing rosewater-and-botanical potion, however, triples as a lip balm, cuticle cream, and "all-around lifesaver," says Fiona Stiles. Just dab it under your eyes to de-puff before applying makeup. Available at DrHauschka.com.

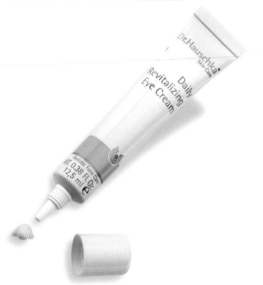

STEAL! The Garnier Nutritioniste Skin Renew Anti-Puff Eye Roller has a cooling metal tip, making application instant and gratifying (and it comes at a more budget-friendly price).

CLINIQUE PORE MINIMIZER INSTANT PERFECTOR

As your skin loses resiliency and starts to sag with age, your pores can appear more pronounced. Enter this mattifying lotion, which eliminates shine and refines the skin's surface, giving the illusion of tightened, smoother skin. It comes in two shades, meaning you'll get the benefit of a little coverage. For best results, apply it to the T-zone before putting on makeup.

STEAL! L'Oreal's Magic Perfecting Base fills in grooves and mattifies and smoothes the skin (though it doesn't come in tinted options like the pricier Clinique product).

LAURA MERCIER TINTED MOISTURIZER SPF 20

Hydrated, even-toned, luminous skin is key to looking like you actually managed a full night's sleep, and this lightweight, award-winning lotion (it's been named an *Allure* Best of Beauty product two years running) delivers on all three counts. It imparts just enough color to offset any sallowness or redness (but it won't appear thick, goopey, or cakey), while providing some UV protection and a hint of shimmer.

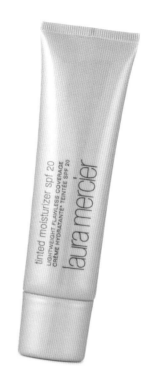

YVES SAINT LAURENT TOUCHE ÉCLAT

Makeup artists, models, and celebrities alike swear by this award-winning golden pen, which is both a magic wand of sorts and the closest thing out there to a "sleep cure"—just a tiny swipe and your tired eyes will go from puffy and red to refreshed. The trick, however, is to use this product less like a concealer and more like a highlighter: apply a little under the brows, to the inner corners of the eyes, along the bridge of your nose, and at the tops of the cheekbones to reflect the light and help your skin look luminous.

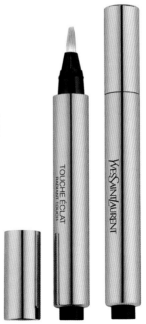

MAC BLOT POWDER

While a matte powder foundation can sap your skin of its youthful glow, this convenient, compact shine buster is great for touch-ups on the go; it absorbs excess oil without leaving a chalky residue.

STEAL! Physician's Formula Mineral Wear Talc-Free Mineral Face Powder absorbs oil without looking dry or Kabuki-cakey, and is gentle enough for breakout-prone or sensitive skin.

JOSIE MARAN CREAM BLUSH IN SUNSET

For a rosy glow, smooth this universally flattering shade on the apples of your cheeks. An added bonus? This lightweight cream is made from all-natural, organic ingredients and contains no parabens, sulfates, or fragrances. Available at Sephora.

ERA RAYZ SPRAY ON BRONZER BY CLASSIFIED COSMETICS

Eradicate that up-all-night-with-newborn pallor! This lightweight spray imparts a sun-kissed glow, and with four shades available—one for fair skin and three for darker complexions—you won't have to worry about telltale orange or too-dark streaks. ("It'll have your friends wondering what desert island you just returned from," says Carmindy.) For a seamless application, aim the spray at a sponge, then rub gently all over your face, making sure it's blended evenly. The spray also works wonders on the décolletage and bare, winter-pale legs. Available at ClassifiedCosmetics.com and Amazon.com.

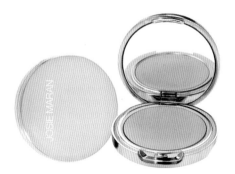

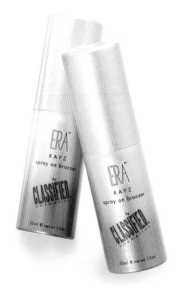

BOBBI BROWN SHIMMER WASH EYE SHADOW

According to Stiles, texture is what you should invest in when choosing an eye shadow, and this sheer, slightly pearlized formula from Bobbi Brown can be used to highlight the brow bone as well as add depth to the lid. Champagne, bronze, and chocolate are universally flattering shades. For a smoky eye, try a shimmery gray or silvery brown, like stone or rock.

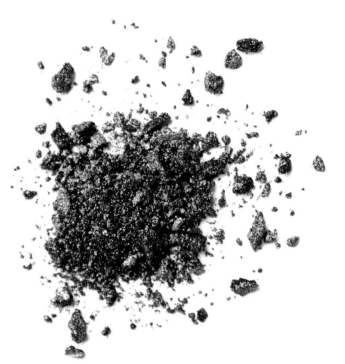

FOREVER STAY EYE PENCIL BY CARMINDY FOR SALLY HANSEN

This waterproof eyeliner may be available for a bargain price (around eight bucks at drugstores), but it glides on like an expensive European product. Perhaps that's because Carmindy had her eponymous makeup line for Sally Hansen produced in Italy, after growing disappointed with formulas she found stateside. "I found that waterproof liners were too soft and didn't deliver enough color, and nonwaterproof formulas smudged too easily," she explains.

To give your eyes a pop, opt for a shade that's opposite your eye color. Try blue if you have brown eyes (and vice versa) or plum if you have green eyes. For hazel eyes, try a jade green. "This is another great way to play up your eyes with minimal makeup—and time!" says Carmindy.

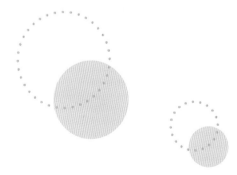

BLINC MASCARA

It's the original tube technology mascara and the gold standard in this category. What it does: Tube technology mascara coats each individual lash in a water-resistant "tube" (as opposed to just painting on color), creating length, lift, volume, and separation without ever clumping, streaking, or flaking. In fact, the makeup comes off *only* when you remove it manually with warm water and gentle pressure. Feel free to wear it at the gym, on a sweltering summer day, to that tearjerker film, or whenever you're feeling hormonal—you won't have to worry about Tammy Faye Bakker eyes, *ever*. Available at boutique beauty stores and spas, Sephora, and blincinc.com.

STEAL! For a less expensive, drugstore equivalent, try L'Oréal Double Extend Beauty Tubes mascara.

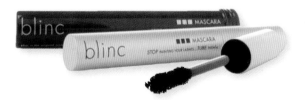

ANASTASIA BROW GEL

Your brows frame your face, which is why anything that better defines and shapes those arches is well worth the investment. And when you're looking for the best in brow control, you go to Anastasia, the makeup maven who built an entire business taming the tiny hairs of celebrities like Madonna, Jennifer Lopez, Penélope Cruz, Naomi Campbell, and Oprah Winfrey. Her eponymous gel is like a clear mascara; use it to brush up and smooth over the brow, giving it shape and uniformity. "Your brows will look groomed no matter how many times you pull a sweater over your head," promises Stiles.

STEAL! For a less expensive version, try LORAC Creamy Brow Pencil, which features a soft pencil tip on one end (to smoothly fill in what nature left out) and a brush on the other to tame unruly hairs. If you live in a very warm climate, you could also check out Make Up For Ever's Waterproof Eyebrow Corrector (available at Sephora). It comes in a tube, but it's easily applied with a brush. Plus, it'll stay put no matter how high the mercury and humidity index rise.

ROSEBUD SALVE

Dry, cracked lips can make you look harried, so banish them with a swipe of this moisturizing balm. Unlike Aquaphor or Vaseline, this cult classic (it comes in a vintage-looking tin) contains a blend of essential oils and cottonseed oil in a base of petrolatum—some even swear by its ability to soothe diaper rash! Available at Sephora, Anthropologie, Urban Outfitters, and Amazon.com. (If you'd prefer not to get your fingertips gooey, try it in tube form or slather on Burt's Bees Beeswax stick in a cool berry tone.)

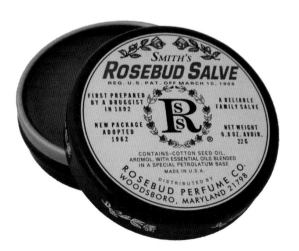

LIPSTICK QUEEN LIPSTICKS AND GLOSSES

Whether you wear lipstick during the day or only at night, you'll find an alluring range of nongreasy, nonsticky textures and colors, including high-shine cherry, velvety berry, and dramatic matte red in this raved-about boutique line. If you're color-shy, stick to a sheer pink—like Jean Queen, which complements most complexions (and most shades of denim). Otherwise, choose a shade that's slightly darker than your skin tone but has peachy undertones (to add warmth and brightness to your face). Available at finer department stores, including Barneys and Henri Bendel, and online at lipstickqueen.com.

STEAL! For beauties on a budget, Stiles says there's no brand with a greater range of shades, textures, and formulations—from the supersaturated ColorBurst lipstick to the more subtle Just Bitten Lipstain + Balm— than Revlon. I am also in love with L'Oréal Infallible lip glosses. They stay on forever and won't dry out your lips. By the way, most drugstores, including CVS and Rite Aid, have a full return policy, great news if you happen to select the wrong shade.

SHISEIDO EYELASH CURLER

L.A. makeup artist Taylor Babaian, who has prettified moms like Mariah Carey and Nelly Furtado, swears by this simple device—and so do I! Curling the lashes makes the eyes look wide open and well rested, and takes almost no time or effort (each eye should take less than 10 seconds). This particular curler is "flatter and wider than other prestige curlers," says Babaian, "which lets you get very close to the base of the lash. The closer you get to the base, the more height you'll get from the lashes." Even better: the edges aren't sharp, so you'll never wince from mistakenly pinching your lids. This is one beauty tool where scrimping just doesn't make sense.

BENEFIT SHE LAQ

This clear liquid sealant helps your carefully applied face stay put and has saved many a mom from raccoon eyes and other makeup mishaps. Apply it over eyeliner, shadow, and brow color and it will prevent pigment from fading, liner from smudging, and shadows and blushes from smearing. The product can be drying, however, so use with caution around the eyes and on sensitive parts of the face—Stiles recommends using waterproof or tube technology mascara instead of applying directly to your lashes.

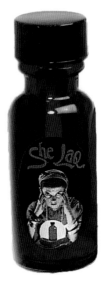

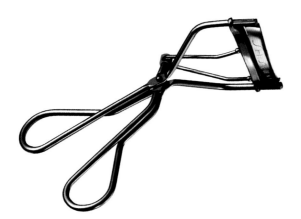

AMLACTIN

Get your tired soles buttery soft with this inexpensive moisturizer, which counts alpha hydroxy acid as one of its star ingredients. "The creamy formula gently exfoliates, replenishes lost moisture, and keeps the surface of your skin looking and feeling smooth," says Dr. Colbert. It's perfect for soothing and smoothing cracked heels or callused fingers, but you can slather it on rough elbows, knees, and ankles, too. Available at drugstores nationwide.

TWEEZERMAN TWEEZERS

The stainless steel Slant tweezers offer the most precise plucking out there thanks to their perfectly angled tips, though you may find yourself using this tool to tame more than just your brows. ("It's unbelievable where you sprout hairs as you get older," confesses Carmindy.) Every mom should have at least two pairs, so there's always one on hand when the other needs sharpening—a service this company provides free of charge.

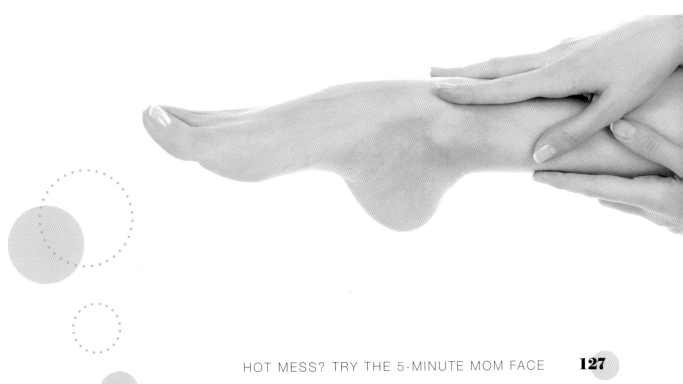

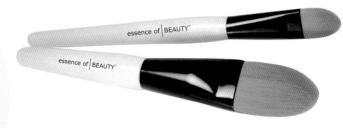

ESSENCE OF BEAUTY MAKEUP BRUSHES

Finding makeup brushes and applicators that don't break down after one use—but don't cost a fortune, either—would typically be a tall order. Makeup artist Carmindy, however, swears by the Essence of Beauty tools, available at CVS pharmacies nationwide: "They are the best inexpensive brushes on the market."

What makes these bargain-priced brushes comparable to more expensive tools from cosmetics companies like MAC or YSL are the high-quality fibers (they don't shed!) as well as the variety of shapes and sizes, which range from a wide Kabuki brush (perfect for mineral makeup and bronzer) to an eye shadow "crease brush" with compact bristles and a slightly rounded center.

3 anti-aging must-haves

"Whenever I drop by Sephora, Barneys, or Walgreens," says dermatologist David Colbert, "I understand why moms are often so perplexed. There are millions of anti-aging products out there. Making the right choice can be daunting." Here, Dr. Colbert helps narrow the market down to these all-you-need essentials.

Retin-A Around the time we hit 40, our collagen and elastin production has slowed down and could benefit from a boost. "Retin-A is one of the few prescription drugs that can actually do this," says Dr. Colbert, "by helping fill in the crevices that develop from the loss of these supporting materials." Since Retin-A can be drying, you'll want to start slowly; apply to the face, neck, and hands only every other evening. Dr. Colbert also suggests following up with a light skin oil to reduce some of the redness and flaking. "Together, these products are like the holy grail of at-home anti-aging treatments."

Hyperpigmentation cream Unsightly brown spots are common signs of age, but they can be treated with gentle bleaching agents, such as kojic acid creams, hydroquinone creams, and glycolic acids. Choosing a lightening cream should be done with the input of your dermatologist, but Dr. Colbert commonly recommends the prescription creams Lustra or Tri-Luma, or kojic acid in serum or cream form (available at drugstores).

A bedtime serum "Our bodies are 60 percent water," says Dr. Colbert. "But when we're sleeping, our bodies become like sponges—they tend to dry out overnight." Drinking a glass or two of water as soon as you get up can help replace some of that lost moisture, but applying a water-based serum before bed is an even better way to keep your skin young and fresh. Look for a serum with hyaluronic acid (which helps hold water in the face), or a combination hyaluronic acid-antioxidant cream—often labeled as vitamin C or vitamin E.

is department store makeup really *better*?

YES and NO According to cosmetic chemist Ni'Kita Wilson, more expensive brands tend to spend more money on ingredients—for example, high-end foundations typically contain better-quality silicones, resulting in a smooth and silky application—but knowing when to save and when to splurge really depends on the category of makeup.

Feel free to scrimp on blush and eyeliner, since on-trend colors often change with the season. Additionally, drugstore biggies like Revlon tend to plow all their R&D funds into lipstick technology, so you might actually benefit from a budget brand more than a designer gloss. And when it comes to mascara, you can't go wrong with a classic tube of Maybelline Great Lash.

Where should you invest? High-end foundations, for one, often impart a more seamless finish than their drugstore counterparts and are typically available in a wider array of color choices and formulations, which makes it easier for you to find the perfect match. Designer eye shadows, too, tend to come in colors that are denser and more saturated, which means they'll stay put longer than some inexpensive brands. Makeup artist Fiona Stiles says that prestige powders are also worth the extra money. "These powders are often more finely pressed and use higher-quality minerals that won't cake or sit on top of your skin."

Just-Right Elegant Evening Makeup

The goal of nighttime makeup isn't to look like you're trying too hard for some kind of Moms Gone Wild outing, but rather, like you're hardly trying. So whether you're primping for an evening out with the girls or date night with your man, choose just *one* feature to highlight with bold, dramatic makeup. Here, makeup artist Carmindy reveals the secrets behind two easy-to-replicate evening looks.

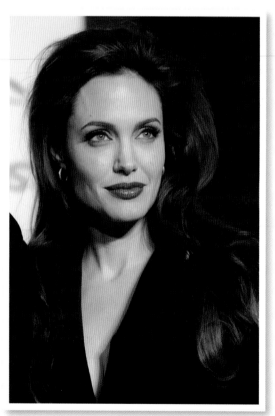

Bold lip: Angelina Jolie

STAR OF THE SHOW: A BOLD, DRAMATIC LIP

Playing up the lips is a great way to get that femme fatale look, *if* you've got a naturally full pout (skip this style if you've got thin lips—a dark gloss will only exaggerate the thinness). Start by lacquering the lips with a shimmery red or berry-tinted gloss (try Chanel Rouge Allure Extrait de Gloss long-wear lip gloss in Excès, Fatale, or Émoi). Then outline the lips and the "V" of the mouth with a highlighting lip liner. (By lining the lips *after* applying color, you'll avoid an overdone matte look.)

SUPPORTING CAST: A NEUTRAL FACE

Dust a shimmery neutral shade across the lids, and line the upper lashes with a chocolate brown pencil. Use a lash curler to help open up the eyes, then add a coat of black mascara.

STAR OF THE SHOW: A SMOKY, SEXY EYE

The secret to perfecting this high-glam look: Start by lining the upper lash line with a black or gray pencil and smudging with an angled eyeliner brush or cotton swab. Then, starting at the lash line, dust a shimmery brown or gray shadow up into the crease, blending the color upward and out. Next, add a lighter shade of shadow (like oatmeal or ivory) underneath the brow bone and to the inner corners of the eyes. To finish, curl the lashes with an eyelash curler and add black mascara.

If you've got a *really* elegant evening planned, there's nothing more glamorous than a few fake lashes. When applied incorrectly, however, falsies can make you look about as demure as a Vegas showgirl. For long, luscious lashes that still look natural, pick up a pack by Ardell (number 110 black), available at drugstores nationwide. When you get home, snip the strip of fake lashes in half (a full set can be cumbersome, says Carmindy) and use only the smaller section. Using just a dab of glue at the seam, place them on the outer corner of the eyes, then sweep a coat of black mascara from root to tip to blend the falsies with the real lashes.

SUPPORTING CAST: A NUDE LIP

You don't want your lips to compete with smoky big browns or baby blues, so add a touch of sheer gloss in a rose-colored hue.

Smoky eye

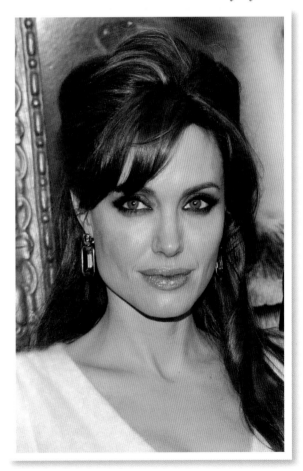

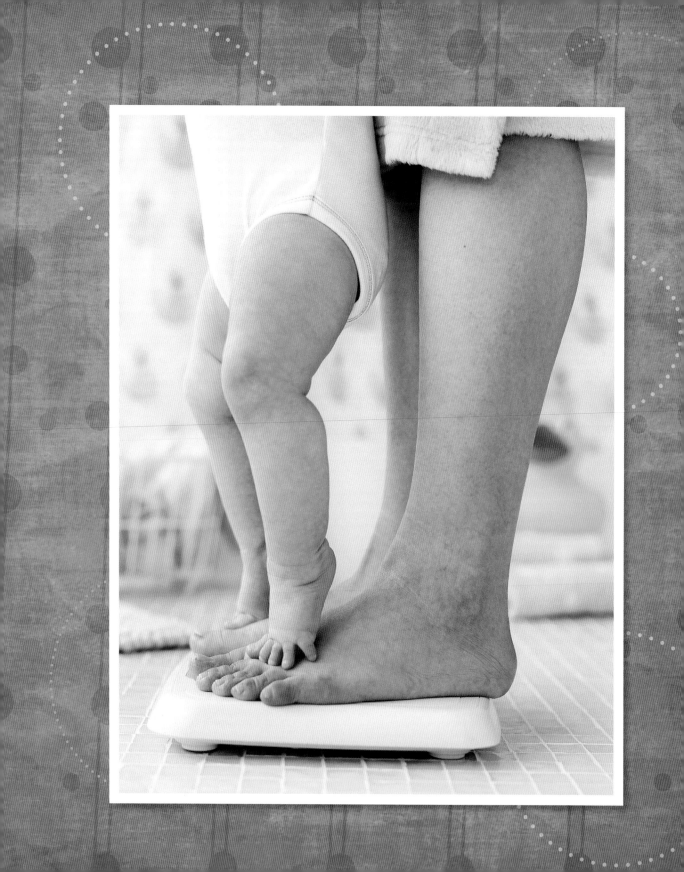

put down those chicken nuggets!

What to Eat (and Avoid) to Get Back into Skinny Jeans

Have you ever been shocked by how often people describe a woman's weight disparagingly, even in the most casual conversations? Like "Oh, you know Sue, that large woman who sits over there," a co-worker might say (about a woman I would never consider large). Or you might hear something like "Whoa, she's a big girl" about someone whom I would never describe as big. A male colleague of mine once commented to me of a female colleague—as she was walking away and possibly still in earshot—"You know, she's fat, but you don't think of her as fat right away because her face isn't fat." Oh. And as someone who lived in New York City for twenty-three years, I can't tell you the number of times I saw a man and woman have a random altercation on the subway or the sidewalk (usually involving personal space issues), and the man would invariably blurt out an insult that would include the word *fat* as a modifier...like "You fat b——" or "If you weren't so fat, there would be room for both of us." Or worse. My takeaways after years of these awful observations are that 1) Anyone not currently in a Victoria's Secret catalog is fair game to be labeled oversize; and 2) Men somehow know that calling a woman "fat" to her face is perhaps the cruelest, worst, and most convenient insult in the world—even when it's coming from a really, really fat guy.

Is it any wonder that so many of us are constantly self-conscious about our bodies, especially after giving birth? We have every media outlet and fashion designer in the world telling us a near anorexic female form is ideal and that there is acclaim to be had if you shed your baby weight quickly (magazine covers! TV reveals! endless compliments!). As celebrity baby mania has swept the country, the obsession with weight has become that much more powerful and pervasive. When I was working at *Us,* it was a sure bet that anytime we ran a "post-baby body" story (and accompanying photo) on our website, it would instantly become a top draw. It didn't matter if it was an überfamous actress or a D-list celebrity hardly anyone's ever heard of, readers clicked on those photos hungrily and rabidly. And it's not just the general public that's driving the trend. Celebrities often stage their own photos to make it *seem* as though they've been "caught" by the paparazzi in a barely there bikini; sometimes they just hire the photographers themselves. It's a way of communicating to the world, "Hey, I'm sexy again. Hire me, Hollywood!" (Most of us had a good laugh whenever staged photos showed up in our in-boxes.)

To top it all off, we live in a society where it's perfectly acceptable to publicly chastise women for their weight. Stars are praised if they don't gain that much weight during pregnancy and lauded for dropping what little weight they do gain within weeks. When they can't (or choose not to), however, they get heckled. Plenty of people snickered when the svelte Kate Hudson gained nearly seventy pounds during her first pregnancy. (When, by the way, did it become okay to criticize *pregnant* women?) These days, postnatal body gazing has evolved into a full-on spectator sport. So somewhere in the back of our minds—when we come home from the hospital with a baby plus thirty extra pounds—we wonder...if thin equals attractive, are we attractive still?

Thus, we drive ourselves crazy. This diet says eat only bacon, this one says to match your diet to your blood type, this one is all about eating foods of the same

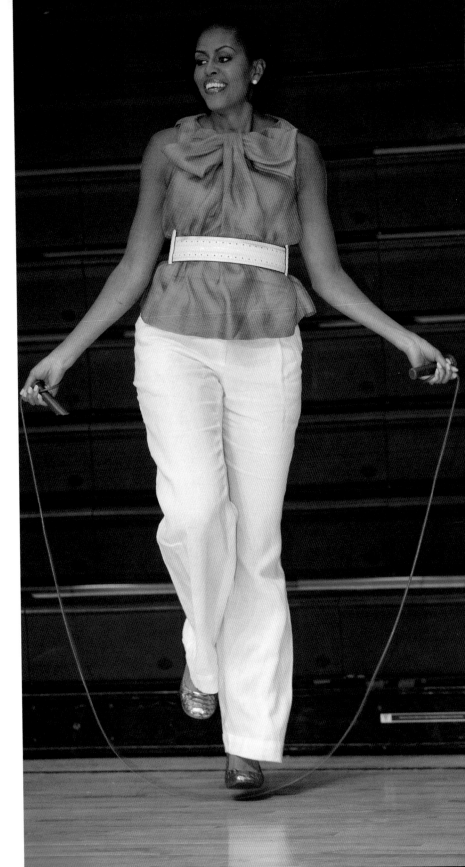

What I'm discovering is the older you get, the more work you have to do to stay there. When I was younger, I could eat whatever I wanted, as long as I exercised; or if I didn't exercise and just watched what I ate, I'd maintain. Well, now I have to do both.
—Michelle Obama

color, and this one is about eating the same things as people in rural Japan. After having covered so many of the diet fads that come and go through celebrity culture, I have learned that every one of them has the same premise—eat less, exercise more—but they're being marketed in different, flashy ways. And we all buy into it.

It wasn't until I had children, however, that I *really* understood just how much misinformation is out there. I was lucky; I didn't really have to worry about my weight as a young adult. In high school I was an avid member of the cross-country team, and I enthusiastically logged mile after mile on the dirt paths near my home in suburban Colorado (and therefore quickly burned off whatever I ate). In fact, one of my fondest memories from that era is running fourteen miles at practice and then coming home and devouring an entire pint of Sara Lee strawberry ice cream—it tasted like heaven. Even in my twenties, my weight never fluctuated much. If I ate a little more than usual for any considerable length of time, I'd hit the gym once or twice and the pounds would melt away. But by the time I turned thirty, things had started to slow down. (It was crushing to realize that, duh, eating ice cream every night really will make you gain weight!) And then, after having my second child at age thirty-six—*boom!*—it was

like my metabolism had suddenly ground to a halt, like some kind of karmic retribution for having been effortlessly thin for so long. Before, I'd always perceived exercise as a free pass to eat pretty much whatever I wanted. Now I was faced with a cold reality: No matter how many downward-facing dogs I might be able to muster, or how much I pretended to enjoy spin class, I wasn't burning off the calories as quickly as I once had. Age and motherhood had caught up to me.

Research tells us that the average adult female will experience anywhere from a 1 to 3 percent reduction in her metabolic rate every year, beginning in her mid-twenties until she levels off somewhere around age fifty. For many of us, that means we're getting pregnant right as our metabolism is slowing from a run to a walk. If you're having children in your forties—and 2008 marked a record number of women over forty doing just that—the struggle to bounce back becomes that much more difficult.

What that all comes down to is this: Exercise is important, but if you want to shed the baby weight, you've got to start seriously watching what you eat. "Baby or no baby," says Hollywood trainer Valerie

Waters, who whipped actresses Jennifer Garner and Poppy Montgomery into postpartum shape, "weight loss is almost always more about the food. Exercise is for making everything else look good."

We all know those mothers who seem to stay thin, no matter how many kids they have or how much they seem to eat. (*So annoying! Seriously.*) For most women, however, weight loss comes slowly and is maintainable only through a healthy, normal relationship with food. In this chapter, I didn't want to present a diet plan per se— contrived diets are short-term solutions (nobody stays on the same "diet" forever) and are often more work than they're worth. Rather, I wanted to cull together all the advice that I wished I had had when I first came home from the hospital—simple, smart strategies to help you cut back calories and avoid weight loss pitfalls. Read on to find out what to eat (and what to avoid) to make it back in your skinny jeans.

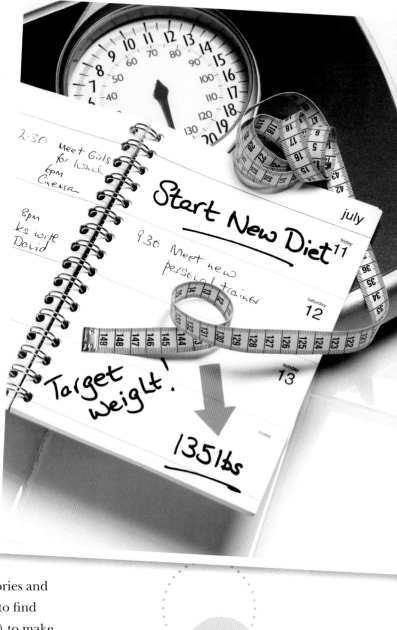

hollywood's biggest losers

Though the recommended weight gain for a pregnant woman of average weight is around twenty-five to thirty-five pounds, sometimes even celebrity moms-to-be overindulge while expecting. (Perhaps that's because, after a life spent dieting to compete for those coveted leading roles, pregnancy offers a bit of a reprieve from counting calories and punishing workouts.) While plenty of A-listers would have you believe that they shed their baby weight overnight with little effort and zero exercise, a precious few have been candid about how much weight they gained and just how much effort it took to lose it.

Kate Hudson

Pregnancy weight gain
65+ pounds (with first baby, Ryder)

How long it took to lose it Ten weeks of three-hour daily workouts (that were so intense, she cried) and a diet of just 1,500 calories a day.

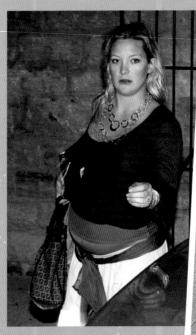

Before

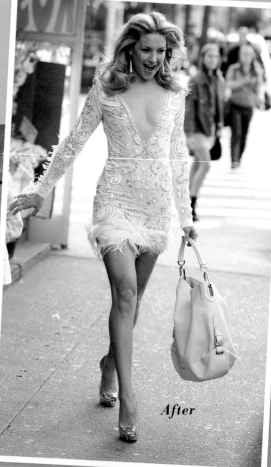

After

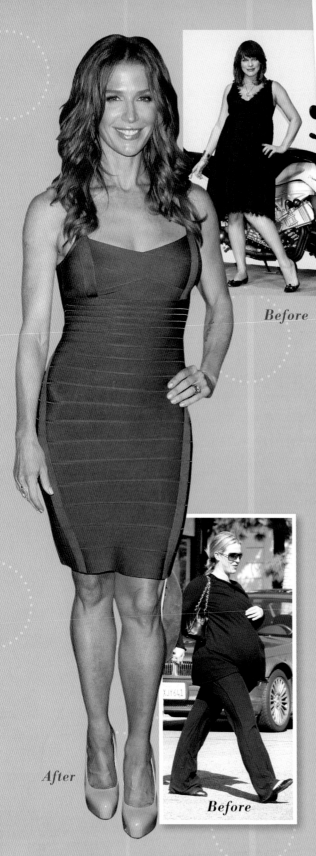

Before

After

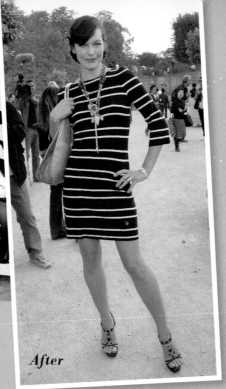

After

Milla Jovovich

Pregnancy weight gain
70+ pounds

How long it took to lose it About a year.
Jovovich slimmed down (losing a majority of the
baby weight in the first five months) thanks to
five-day-a-week workouts with celebrity trainer
Harley Pasternak and a meal delivery service.

Poppy Montgomery

Pregnancy weight gain
70+ pounds

How long it took to lose it Around nine months.
The *Without a Trace* star worked out six days
a week (she's a fan of P90X fitness DVDs) and
limited herself to just 1,200 calories a day.

Before

9 Ways We Self-Sabotage Our Diet

Most of us already understand the basics of healthy eating—we know, of course, that a mixed greens salad with vinaigrette is better than a burger, that steamed veggies have fewer calories than a side of mashed potatoes, that birthday cake isn't exactly something you should eat for breakfast. It's not that we don't understand nutrition or that we can't differentiate between a healthy snack and a fatty treat. We struggle because our schedules are crazy and jam-packed, because we're often more concerned with feeding our kids than feeding ourselves, and because we unwittingly self-sabotage. We tell ourselves that just *one* bite of mac and cheese "won't really matter" or that certain calories "just don't count."

How many times have you picked at your kids' leftover plain pasta with butter *before* sitting down to dinner yourself? Or just *had* to have a frothy Frappuccino because you were falling asleep by midafternoon? Or totally forgot about that handful or two (or *three!*) of Teddy Grahams you ate— straight from the box—while cleaning up the kitchen? Recent studies show that we all underestimate how many calories we're actually consuming. So if you're not shedding the pounds, you can bet that

you're taking in more calories than you think. Following are the most common reasons new moms can't seem to slim down, plus advice to help you break the cycle.

WE HAVE NO IDEA HOW MUCH WE'RE EATING

One of the easiest strategies for losing weight is to keep a food journal—that is, to make a written note of every single morsel of food you eat as soon as it goes in your mouth. Carrie Underwood successfully implemented this technique in her quest to slim down after winning *American Idol* (she eventually shaved twenty pounds off her five-foot-three-inch frame). Out of curiosity, I thought I'd try it, too, even though it seemed like just one more thing to do (and also kind of weirdly obsessive). But after just a few days, I admit I was shocked to see how much I was really eating. One day I realized that I'd put down nearly three thousand calories; the next day, it wasn't until I looked at my notes that I remembered I'd had a midmorning cookie. Writing it down keeps you accountable. I guarantee that if you knew you'd already eaten two thousand

true or false?

The Master Cleanse and other detox diets can help you drop pounds fast like celebrities do.

TRUE...and FALSE No doubt you've heard plenty of celebrities swear that some juice fast or detox diet helped them shed extra weight and squeeze into a slinky designer dress. Sarah Jessica Parker, for example, is a fan of the BluePrintCleanse, Beyoncé claimed to have lost twenty pounds on the Master Cleanse (a concoction of fresh lime or lemon juice, maple syrup, and cayenne pepper mixed with water, consumed six to twelve times a day), and Gwyneth Paltrow once posted her own plan for a seven-day fast on her website, GOOP. It's no wonder almost every mom I know is dying to try one—the stars make these "miracle diets" seem so easy. But the question is: Do they really work?

In the short term, you absolutely will lose weight—cleanses and detox diets emphasize extreme calorie reduction (in its most generous program, the BluePrintCleanse delivers just 1,070 calories a day). "All 'detox' diets will lead to weight loss because they are so low in calories," confirms nutritionist and creator of the F-Factor Diet Tanya Zuckerbrot. "However,

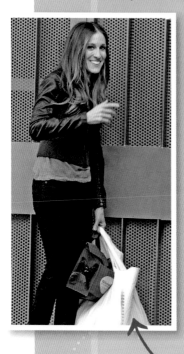

cleanses are temporary solutions and they're probably the worst thing you can do for your body; weight loss needs to occur over time."

What's that, you say? The *worst* thing you can do? That's because fasts may help you shed pounds in the short term, but they're practically a guarantee that you'll gain weight—perhaps even more than you lost in the first place—as soon as you reintroduce normal food into your diet. Because let's face it: If you've been starving yourself for a week, you'll be that much more likely to break the fast with a juicy steak, fries, and a hunk of cheesecake. There's also little evidence to support the notion that detox diets actually help remove any "toxins" that have built up in the body.

Several years ago, a young woman in my office decided to try a cleanse. Once bubbly and energetic, she morphed within days into someone glassy-eyed and listless. Personally, I can't imagine trying to be an effective parent when you're so hungry that you're about to chew off your own arm. A healthy diet in tandem with consistent exercise is still the best (and certainly safest) option to lose the baby weight. Save the cleanses for the celebrities—and don't even *think* about trying one if you're still breastfeeding.

Sarah Jessica Parker has used the BluePrintCleanse.

calories by lunch, you'd be more likely to eat a lighter supper. (By the way, I never kept up the food journal but it was a good experiment in being mindful.)

WE THINK BREAST-FEEDING IS THE SECRET TO WEIGHT LOSS

Almost every celeb mom—from Angelina Jolie to Kelly Preston to Naomi Watts to Heidi Klum—has attributed her rapid postbirth weight loss to breastfeeding. While it's true that breastfeeding burns an average of five hundred extra calories a day, not every woman will see the difference when it comes to her waistline. "About half of women will swear that breastfeeding helped them lose weight, and the other half will blame breastfeeding for keeping them from their weight loss goals," says Dr. Shari Brasner.

Adds trainer Valerie Waters: "Just because an actor in a magazine or your sister or your best friend lost the weight super quickly while nursing doesn't mean it's going to happen that way for you. It's a myth to think that we all lose weight the same way. Everyone's body is different; I've actually had clients who didn't lose those last few pounds until they *stopped* nursing."

It's important to remember just how little five hundred extra calories a day really is—don't think you can keep "eating for two." At the same time, no woman should "diet" (read: drastically restrict her caloric intake) while breastfeeding. Instead, focus on making healthy choices when it comes to what you're eating and keeping your weight-loss goals realistic.

WE DRINK OURSELVES FAT

It seems crazy to think that something so innocent as a midday coffee break or a post-exercise thirst quencher could actually be one of the reasons you can't seem to shed the baby weight. However, countless studies have shown not only that the average portion size of most soft drinks has grown considerably in the last few decades, but that high-calorie beverages may be one of the leading causes of widespread obesity in this country. Just because it comes in a bottle or a can doesn't mean the calories don't count. Sugar mixed with water comes in many forms and under many labels (even those purporting to have health benefits). Are you sabotaging your slim-down with these liquid diet busters?

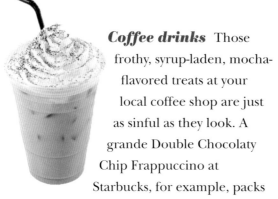

Coffee drinks Those frothy, syrup-laden, mocha-flavored treats at your local coffee shop are just as sinful as they look. A grande Double Chocolaty Chip Frappuccino at Starbucks, for example, packs 500 calories and *98 grams of carbs*—that's nearly the same amount of carbohydrates as a large chili, a baked potato, and a side salad with ranch dressing from Wendy's, or a Big Country Breakfast Platter from Hardee's. If you really need the midday creamy caffeine boost, try a grande caffè latte with 2 percent milk (190 calories) or skim milk (130 calories). And seriously, skip the whipped cream.

Sports drinks If you've managed to get in a workout, don't negate the benefits by chugging a "sports drink." Beverages like Gatorade and Powerade (which can pack more than 300 calories per bottle) were formulated to replace the electrolytes lost by rigorous exercise—like playing a four-hour professional football game or running a marathon, not logging twenty minutes on the elliptical. If you're seriously craving the sweetness or just find water too boring, try diluting sports drinks by at least 50 percent or choosing a low- or no-calorie variety.

Cocktails You've been with the kids all week, you finally booked a sitter, and you've got a chance to gossip with the girls over dinner or unwind with your man on date night. Go ahead and have a drink (or two). Just keep in mind that boozing it up can undo all that careful calorie counting. Among the worst offenders? The mai tai (at 620 calories for a 9-ounce drink), the piña colada (586 calories per 12 ounces), the margarita (550 calories per 10 ounces), and the Long Island iced tea (543 calories per 10 ounces). Just to put that in context, a McDonald's Big Mac packs 540 calories. Pass on frozen, sugar-filled cocktails and opt for one of these drinks that won't derail your diet:

Single shot of vodka with club soda or Sprite Zero	65 calories*
Glass of chardonnay or cabernet sauvignon	90 calories
Champagne	90 calories
Mimosa	75 calories
Rum and Diet Coke	65 calories
Gin and diet tonic	65 calories
Martini, shaken with ice and a splash of vermouth	160 calories
Light beer	110 calories

Calories estimated by Calwineries.com

WE EAT OFF OUR KIDS' PLATES

I know that nearly every parenting expert on the planet will preach the importance of eating dinner together as a family, but sometimes that's just not feasible or—let's face it—even desirable. (At some point, we could all use a grown-up meal and some adult conversation...after the kids have gone to bed.) Most moms, then, end up in a familiar scenario: While rushing to feed the children by five-thirty P.M., you start to feel a little hungry—suddenly, you're shoveling in a few forkfuls of mac and cheese while standing over the kitchen sink. Or, for those working mothers among us, you rush home from the office just as the kids are pushing away a half-finished plate of finger food, and you start absentmindedly picking at whatever might be left over.

The problem with this kind of mindless eating is that the extra calories add up fast. "You can easily rack up an extra three hundred to five hundred calories a day from nibbling at dinner. *Easily,*" says nutritionist Keri Glassman, who has worked with hot mom Jennifer Lopez. That's enough to sabotage your efforts at shedding the pounds and enough to render your evening jog or morning spin class practically null and void. To avoid this kind

of temptation, Glassman recommends two dinnertime strategies:

1. Make "kid food" your main meal If you really want to nibble on chicken nuggets and French fries, order or make them for yourself—and call that dinner. "This attitude of, 'Oh, I'm just having a bite,' doesn't work," says Glassman. If you actually have to choose between eating an appetizing "grown-up" meal and eating a plate of chicken nuggets, chances are you'll hold out for something better.

2. Fill up on healthy snacks Stock the house with almost-no-calorie snacks to tide you over until dinner. "Moms are often busy preparing their kids' meals before they've had a chance to eat themselves," Glassman explains. *Of course* you're hungry. Munching on a guilt-free treat, like cucumber salad, red peppers with salsa, carrot sticks and hummus, or endive leaves, or sipping a cup of herbal tea can help curb your cravings.

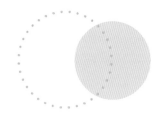

how just a few nibbles a day can add up to major weight gain

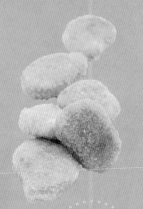

2 chicken nuggets (93 calories)

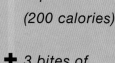

+ 10 French fries (15 calories each; 150 calories total)

+ half a juice box (6.8 ounces; 47 calories)

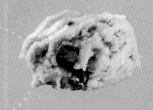

+ spoonful of cookie dough (70 calories)

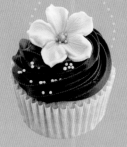

+ 1 birthday cupcake (200 calories)

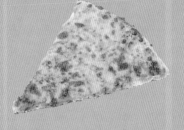

+ 3 bites of cheese pizza (83 calories)

= 643 calories

WE MAKE VERY BAD CHOICES WHEN DINING OUT

When was the last time you ate a plate of fried calamari at home before digging in to your main course? It's no secret that the social aspects of dining out lend themselves to three-course meals and indulgent desserts—not to mention the fact that restaurant portions are huge, and they're typically loaded with salt, fat, sugar, and butter. (They've got to make it taste good so we'll keep coming back!) Eating out can be perilous when you're trying to slim down. In fact, a study conducted at the University of Texas at Austin found that dieters ate an average of 240 more calories on days they dined at a restaurant. (Frankly, I think that seems like kind of a lowball estimate.) Instead of vowing never to dine out again, however, consider the following strategies suggested by nutritionist Tanya Zuckerbrot to make the experience less catastrophic:

Start with a soup or salad Clear, broth-based soups (like miso, minestrone, and chicken vegetable) and salads with oil and vinegar dressing on the side are low-calorie options. "Start with these and you'll be less likely to dig into the bread basket or the fried appetizers on the table," says Zuckerbrot.

Scan the menu for key words When it comes to your entrée, look for words like grilled, broiled, steamed, or roasted; these selections will have fewer calories than pan-seared or fried options.

Skip the starch Many entrées come with a side of pasta, rice, or a baked potato as well as a vegetable. Ask for a double portion of vegetables instead.

Always order dressing and sauces on the side Eliminate high-fat sauces and dressing (like honey-mustard, blue cheese, and ranch), or order them on the side and use them sparingly—try dipping just the tip of your fork in the sauce rather than the entire bite of food. And it doesn't hurt to request that little or no oil be used to cook your entrée. "Some people are embarrassed to make these kinds of requests," says Zuckerbrot. "Don't be." After all, you're paying for the meal.

Follow the three-bite rule When it comes to desserts, studies show that people always rate the first and last bites as the best. "Three bites gives you a first, middle, and last, which is all you need to appreciate a sweet treat," says Zuckerbrot. Ordering a cup of coffee or tea at meal's end can help you resist the urge to eat the entire slice of cake or pie.

what to eat when eating out: the best restaurant options

Olive Garden's Venetian Apricot Chicken

This lighter selection of grilled chicken breast in an apricot-citrus sauce, paired with broccoli, asparagus, and diced tomatoes, is a low-fat option that's big on flavor. "There are only 380 calories in the entire dish," says Zuckerbrot. "Plus, you'll get 8 grams of fiber."

P.F. Chang's Asian Grilled Norwegian Salmon on brown rice

(from the lunch menu). This salmon dish has 320 calories per serving and—when compared with most other restaurant fare—is relatively low in sodium.

Romano's Macaroni Grill Jumbo Shrimp Rosemary Spiedini

Steer clear of heavy, creamy pasta dishes and opt instead for this guilt-free dish with roasted vegetables—just 300 calories.

Outback Steakhouse Grilled Chicken on the Barbie & Fresh Seasonal Mixed Veggies

Skip the butter and this fill-you-up dish comes in at just over 400 calories.

Wendy's large chili and side salad

One of the better fast-food options. The large chili has 280 calories and 7 grams of fiber, while a side salad with mandarin oranges and half a fat-free dressing pack has 150 calories and 4 grams of fiber.

WE DRINK DIET SODA

Most of us feel pretty good about ourselves whenever we choose a Diet Coke over the real thing. After all, there are zero calories in diet soda. Surely the diet drink is a responsible choice, right? Unfortunately, your faux sugar habit may be sabotaging your quest to slim down.

Diet soda on its own won't cause any weight gain (again, diet sodas have zero calories). However, diet sodas are loaded with artificial sweeteners, which may lead to cravings for other forms of sugar, "and that *can* lead to weight gain," says Zuckerbrot. In fact, recent research has suggested that the more diet sodas a person drinks, the more likely he or she is to pack on the pounds. While scientists still don't know exactly why that is yet, it's possible that some people feel as though they've earned a "pass" by choosing a diet drink and therefore don't feel the need to restrict calories elsewhere; others believe artificial sweeteners may create a craving for sugar that ultimately goes unfulfilled. (I know I sometimes crave something sweet, like a cookie or brownie, while drinking a diet soda.) Artificial sweeteners may also cause bloat and gas (like you need your stomach to be any poochier, right?), and the caffeine can trigger a midday crash.

If you're having trouble kicking the soda habit, try squeezing some fresh limes or lemons into a pitcher of sparkling water; you'll still get the fizz without all the fake sugar.

WE STOCK THE FRIDGE WITH JUNK

Keeping your fridge chock-full of unhealthy, fatty foods is like giving an alcoholic (or a teenager) the key to your liquor cabinet—it's a temptation too strong to resist. So the same rule you might apply to your kids should work for you, too: If you don't want them to eat it, don't keep it in the house. And remember, it won't be long before your kids are rummaging through the fridge all on their own, if they aren't already. Would you rather they reach for an apple and yogurt or chug a can of soda and throw a Hot Pocket in the microwave? "It's not too early to think that your baby or young children are going to see what you are eating and learn your habits," adds Glassman. "You'll want them to be eating real meals, too."

So, what to toss? Check out the pictures (next page) and then keep reading.

BAD FRIDGE

GOOD FRIDGE

Frozen veggies make a healthy side dish in little to no time.

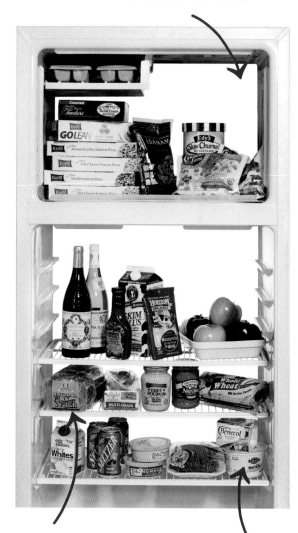

Toss the sodas and soft drinks.

Creamy salad dressings are a common source of "hidden" calories.

Swap butter for a low-fat, nondairy spread.

Whole grains have more nutrients than white bread.

Choose low-sugar, high protein Greek yogurt over the processed pink stuff.

TOSS! *Processed, packaged foods and refined grains* When it comes to selecting healthy foods, there's a general rule of thumb: The closer the food is to the way it exists in nature, the better it is for you. When you're biting into an apple, for example, it's the same fruit that grew on a tree somewhere; it hasn't been injected with preservatives or sodium, hasn't been fried or frozen, hasn't been stripped of its natural nutrients. Heavily processed and packaged foods, on the other hand, are loaded with artificial ingredients, fats, salts, sugars, and preservatives so they'll stay "fresh" on the shelf at the store. The same holds true for refined grains; foods like white rice, white bread, and puffed cereal have been stripped of their natural nutrients. Whenever possible, choose foods in their "natural" state—fresh fruits and vegetables, unrefined grains (like brown or wild rice and 100 percent whole-grain bread), and lean meats and proteins. The fewer processed foods in your fridge, the better.

TOSS! *"Low-fat" or "no-fat" foods* Be wary of anything labeled low-fat or no-fat. Marketers are smart; they know consumers will be inclined to reach for a low-fat option because it seems like the healthier choice. But low-fat and no-fat foods often have very high sugar and

sodium content, to hide the fact that there's not much fat (and not much flavor). Just because the package says "low-fat" doesn't mean it's good for you—or your waistline. Too much sodium can make you bloat, while too much sugar—especially fructose—has been linked to increased abdominal fat. Also, steer clear of commercial salad dressings, low-fat or otherwise, in favor of extra-virgin olive oil and a splash of vinegar. The majority of commercial salad dressings are filled with sodium, high-fructose corn syrup, and various preservatives. Before you know it, you've turned a healthy green salad into a hidden calorie trap.

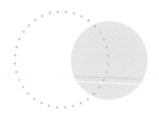

true or false?

You'll gain weight if you eat after 8 P.M.

FALSE The reason so many people think eating at night causes weight gain is that we tend to eat *extra* at night, without accounting for what we've already eaten earlier in the day (we're also more likely to reach for unhealthy snacks and mindlessly put away several hundred calories while sitting glassy-eyed in front of the television). The truth is that the more calories you eat, the more weight you gain—regardless of when you consume those calories. It all comes down to calories in versus calories out.

true or false?

Spicy foods can make you skinny.

TRUE-*ish* Capsaicin, the active component in chili peppers, creates a burning sensation when it comes into contact with human tissues (which is why you'll find it in many pain and anti-itch medications as well as muscle-soothing creams). The heat that's generated by *eating* spicy foods triggers a temporary boost in your metabolic rate—probably not enough to actually burn any more calories, but enough to help briefly suppress your appetite, according to recent research. "Spicy foods make you feel fuller and, therefore, you consume less actual food," says Zuckerbrot. "Perhaps that's why some of the healthiest ethnic diets are Thai, Vietnamese, and Indian." Consider adding a little heat to your next meal with red pepper flakes or jalapeños—skip the processed hot sauce, however, which is most likely loaded with artificial ingredients, salt, and preservatives.

WE GET OVERWHELMED IN THE GROCERY STORE

The average American supermarket carries nearly forty thousand items, so it's easy to get overwhelmed (and to toss lots of high-sugar, high-fat junk in your cart because it looks so tantalizing). Instead of getting bogged down perusing the latest processed snack foods and frozen entrées, shop for easy-to-prepare ingredients that can be thrown together without much fuss. Frozen veggies, for example, can be sautéed for a quick and healthy side dish. A small handful of dried fruit and unsalted nuts makes a filling grab-and-go snack. (And a George Foreman makes grilling up any kind of lean protein—from chicken sausage to fish filets to turkey burgers—a snap.) Next time you head to the supermarket, fill your cart with these simple-to-use staples recommended by Zuckerbrot and Glassman.

Cereals

Plain (meaning nonflavored) microwavable oatmeal packets
Fiber One, Original
All-Bran Original
All-Bran Bran Buds

Breads and Crackers

GG Scandinavian Bran Crispbread
Thomas' Light Multi-Grain English Muffins
100% whole-grain bread
Boboli 100% Whole Wheat or Tabula Rasa (Trader Joe's brand) Whole Grain Pizza Crust

Pasta and Rice

Texmati brown rice or Uncle Ben's Fast & Natural Whole Grain Instant Brown Rice (cooks in 10 minutes!)
Barilla Plus or Ronzoni Healthy Harvest whole-grain pasta

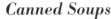

Canned Soups

Progresso Vegetable Classics garden vegetable soup
Amy's Lentil, Fat-free Chunky Vegetable, and Low-Fat Minestrone

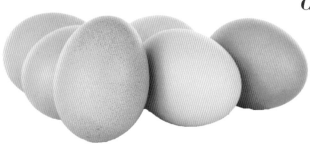

Meats

Tuna fish canned in water

Lean cold cuts: turkey, chicken, ham, or roast beef

Boneless, skinless chicken breast

Turkey or chicken sausage

Lean cuts of beef, pork, lamb, and fish

Dairy

Eggs

Fage Total 0% yogurt

Laughing Cow Light cheese

Low-sodium cottage cheese (such as Friendship 1% Lowfat No Salt Added)

Skim, soy, or almond milk

Fruits & Vegetables

Any and all (except starchy veggies like potatoes and corn)

Frozen Foods

Frozen vegetables

Edamame

Frozen berries

General Grocery

Polaner Sugar Free Preserves with Fiber

Smucker's Low Sugar and Sugar Free variety jams

Marinara sauce (with no sugar added)

Any of Whole Foods' 365 Everyday Value pasta sauces

All natural peanut butter (no sugar added)

Assorted nuts (almonds, pecans, walnuts) with no salt added

Assorted dried fruit (cranberries, cherries, blueberries) with no sugar added

Low-sodium salsa

Sabra classic hummus

Extra-virgin olive oil

White wine vinegar

Snack Foods

Gnu Flavor & Fiber Bar

Fiber One 90-calorie bars

Air-popped popcorn (like Orville Redenbacher's SmartPop! mini bags or Jolly Time Healthy Pop minis)

Desserts and Chocolate

Tofutti pops or some other sugar-free, fat-free fudge pops

Sugar-free Jell-O

Kozy Shack No Sugar Added Chocolate pudding

Skinny Cow chocolate truffle bar

Keebler Right Bites Fudge Shoppe Mini Fudge Stripes 100-calorie packs

Naturally sweet herbal teas

WE CAN'T DECIDE WHAT'S FOR DINNER

If you're anything like me, the real difficulty with sticking to a "diet" or just eating well isn't avoiding the candy aisle at the supermarket; it's figuring out what to do with all those healthy foods once you get them home. (After a crazy workday and time shuttling the kids around, the thought of playing Jamie Oliver at home—no matter how many fruits and vegetables are stuffed in my refrigerator—is really not appealing.) At right, you'll find a mix & match–style meal plan—a week's worth of breakfast, lunch, dinner, and snack ideas—featuring only the foods from the shopping list on pages 152–153. Everything is super-simple to prepare, so no matter how hectic your day has been (or how tired you actually are), you'll have an answer next time you hear, "Hey, Mom, what's for dinner?"

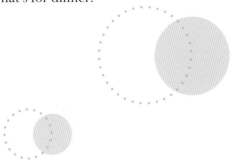

MONDAY

Breakfast Cereal with low-fat or skim milk + any fruit (like mixed berries or half a grapefruit) + coffee or tea (no added sugar)

Snack Laughing Cow Light cheese and GG Scandinavian Bran Crispbread crackers

Lunch Tuna packed in water + mixed greens salad + any veggies of your choice + olive oil and vinegar dressing

Snack Air-popped popcorn

Dinner Grilled chicken sausage with sautéed frozen vegetables (throw the sausage on a George Foreman grill and the veggies in a pan—ridiculously simple)

Dessert Fat-free, sugar-free fudge pop

TUESDAY

Breakfast 2 eggs (prepared however you like) + whole-grain toast + any fruit + coffee or tea (no added sugar)

Snack Fiber One 90-calorie bar

Lunch Soup + mixed greens salad

Snack Edamame

Dinner Baked or roasted boneless, skinless chicken breasts (marinate first with a little olive oil, fresh lemon juice, and a sprig of rosemary for a kick of flavor) + any vegetable

Dessert Sugar-free Jell-O

WEDNESDAY

Breakfast Greek yogurt + mixed berries + coffee or tea (no added sugar)

Snack Dried fruit + nuts

Lunch Turkey, roast beef, or ham sandwich on whole-grain bread with mustard, lettuce, and tomato + Laughing Cow Light cheese + a handful of grapes

Snack Red peppers and low-sodium salsa

Dinner Whole-wheat pasta + marinara sauce + small mixed greens salad

Dessert Herbal tea

THURSDAY

Breakfast Oatmeal + any fruit + coffee or tea (no sugar added)

Snack Cucumber slices dressed in olive oil and balsamic vinegar

Lunch Soup

Snack Edamame

Dinner Steak stir-fry with frozen veggies and brown rice (these days, you can get the health benefits of brown rice with the speed of an instant variety!)

Dessert Keebler Right Bites Fudge Shoppe Mini Fudge Stripes

FRIDAY

Breakfast Low-sodium cottage cheese + fruit of your choice + coffee or tea (no sugar added)

Snack Fiber One 90-calorie bar

Lunch Tuna packed in water + mixed greens salad + any veggies of your choice + olive oil and vinegar dressing

Snack Endive leaves + hummus

Dinner Whole-wheat, pre-made pizza crust + marinara sauce + veggies of your choice + a sprinkle of low-fat mozzarella

Dessert Skinny Cow chocolate truffle bar or Kozy Shack Chocolate pudding

SATURDAY

Breakfast English muffin + all-natural peanut butter + coffee or tea (no sugar added)

Snack Greek yogurt + mixed berries

Lunch Turkey, roast beef, or ham sandwich on whole-grain bread with mustard, lettuce, and tomato + Laughing Cow Light cheese + a handful of grapes

Snack Air-popped popcorn

Dinner Baked or grilled salmon + steamed veggies of your choice + mixed greens salad

Dessert Sugar-free Jell-O

SUNDAY

Breakfast 2 egg omelet (add frozen vegetables) + whole-grain toast + coffee or tea (no sugar added)

Snack Dried fruit + nuts

Lunch Soup

Snack Carrot sticks + hummus

Dinner Turkey burger + steamed vegetable of your choice + mixed greens salad

Dessert Fat-free, sugar-free fudge pop

10 ways to stop feeling hungry

Don't clean your plate Although many of us were raised to do just that, studies have shown that portion sizes have increased dramatically in the last few decades. There's no reward—except for extra pounds—in being a member of the Clean Plate Club. Besides, forcing yourself to eat an arbitrary amount of food (that is, whatever you threw on the plate) messes with your ability to determine when you're really full and when you're eating just because you feel you should.

Never eat straight from the carton Glassman says putting your food on a plate will help you visualize just how much you're really eating—it's too easy to overeat if you're munching mindlessly from a bag of chips or eating straight from the take-out box.

Get out of the house The more time you spend out and about, the less you'll be tempted to eat the food that's piled up in your pantry, says celebrity trainer Ramona Braganza.

Have a cup of tea or a glass of water with every meal It will help fill you up, as well as help you eat more slowly.

Eat a balanced breakfast Research shows that people who do are up to 50 percent less likely to become obese; breakfast staves off the need to snack and indulge in oversize meals later in the day.

Downsize your dishware There's truth to the notion that your eyes may often be bigger than your stomach. Studies show that people tend to consume more food when eating off larger plates and out of larger bowls.

Eat before you go out Whether you're attending a wedding, a baby shower, a holiday brunch, or a birthday party, you're more likely to overdo it at the buffet line if you arrive starving or if no healthy food options are being served. Eat a light, low-calorie snack before you go; it'll help you avoid temptation.

Don't eat in front of the television It's distracting, and you'll likely overeat.

Brush your teeth The morning (or evening) brush-and-floss routine signals to your body that you've finished eating. Plus, orange juice—and just about all other foods—tastes terrible once you've brushed.

Healthy snacks should contain protein *and* fiber The combo will keep you feeling fuller longer, as well as keep your blood sugar stable (so you won't have that midday crash to contend with). Try mozzarella cheese and apple slices, unsalted nuts with dried fruit, or veggie slices and hummus.

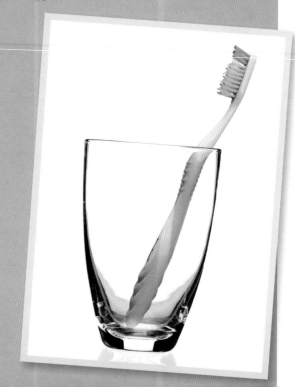

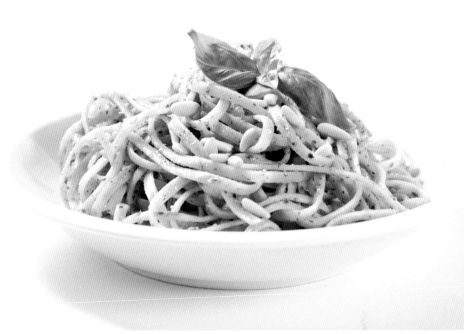

true or false?

Carbohydrates will make you fat.

FALSE It's one of the biggest diet myths out there, thanks largely to the no-carb craze and the popularity of programs like Atkins and the South Beach Diet. But it's the quantity we eat that packs on the pounds. For example, "Italians live on pasta," says Zuckerbrot, "but they eat pasta as a first course, limiting their servings to about one cup, or 375 calories. Then they eat a main course of lean meat or fish and vegetables. In America, we often eat pasta as our main course, which is about four cups, or 1,000 calories. Big difference!"

While carbs themselves won't necessarily cause you to gain weight, it is a good idea to trade in unrefined carbs (like white bread and white pasta) for refined varieties (like whole-grain bread and whole-wheat pasta). Whole, unrefined grains have more nutrients and more fiber than their refined, processed counterparts and thus don't convert to sugar as quickly.

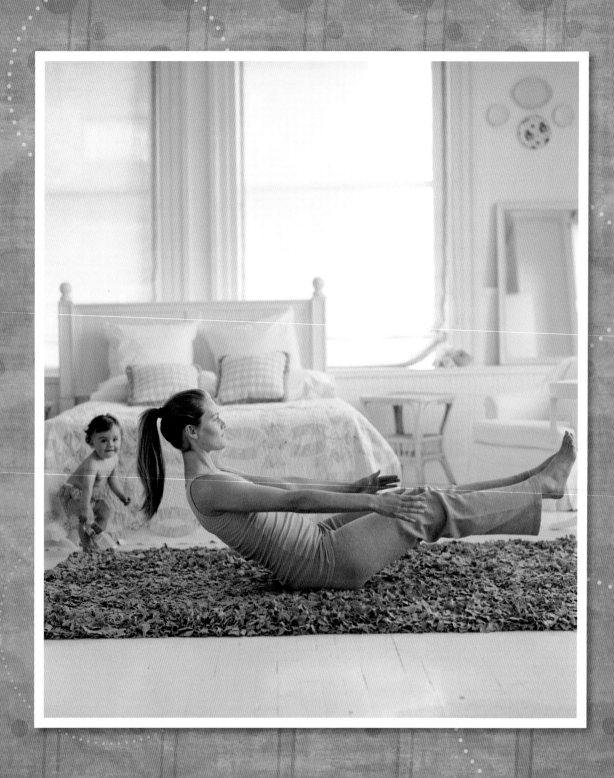

it's never too late to shed the baby weight

Whether Your Child Is 6 Months or 16 Years

I learned nearly everything about the ways that certain celebrities live their lives while I was working at *Us Weekly*. And it's always amazed me just how much information *doesn't* make it out there (certainly we didn't publish a good deal of it) and how much society can be fooled by some of these fabulous famous people. Just as there were people who were shocked— *shocked,* I tell you—when, say, Ricky Martin came out of the closet or Pam Anderson and Kid Rock filed for divorce, there are those who can't quite fathom the kinds of shortcuts some celebrities take to get thin. There are stars who abuse the attention deficit drug Adderall to stay slim, some who purge regularly in nightclub bathrooms, those who get their breasts done multiple times, and others who get lipo as often as most people go to the dentist. Those stars who say they eat tons of bacon cheeseburgers? Probably not. And those who say they hate working out and never do it probably work out every day. When it comes to glam shots—forget it; almost all of them are retouched. Arms are thinned out, waists pinched, thighs shaved, and wrinkles erased. For red carpet events and photo shoots, nearly all the stars will sport (ridiculously expensive) hair extensions, so not even those gorgeous, flowing locks are signs of natural-born beauty. Still, we all try to measure up to these impossible-to-achieve standards and feel pretty awful about ourselves when we can't.

Let's get serious: Most of us will *never* look like Angelina Jolie or Adriana Lima or any of those celeb moms with impossibly perfect physiques. In fact, comparing yourself with any woman—whether she's famous or not—isn't realistic, isn't really fair, and is certainly not helpful. (If you didn't look like Jennifer Lopez before you got pregnant, why would you beat yourself up for not looking like her *after* having a baby?!) If it were your full-time job to look as gorgeous and glamorous as possible— and you had all the money in the world at your disposal—you could probably look like an A-list star, too. But this is real life. At some point, we have to stop the madness and start aiming for goals that are actually attainable. You may not be able to mimic Kelly Ripa's taut tummy (I think she might be a genetic aberration), but you *can* tone flabby arms, lift and firm the booty, and trim inches off your waist. What it takes to do that isn't magic; it's a better diet and dedicated work in the gym. Jessica Alba once said her post-baby workouts were so intense, she cried. And after giving birth to her first daughter, Jennifer Garner admitted to *People* magazine that it wasn't until she got serious about working out that she was able to shed the pounds: "It took me a long, long time. I just wasn't that motivated. I wanted to play with her. Then I got on the treadmill, stopped stuffing my face, and lost the weight."

A HISTORY OF THE HOT MOM PHENOM

1967 MILF enters the mainstream? Anne Bancroft—aka Mrs. Robinson— seduces Dustin Hoffman in *The Graduate,* wearing nothing more than lacy black lingerie and heels.

1991 A pregnant Demi Moore sparks huge controversy by posing nude on the cover of *Vanity Fair's* August issue.

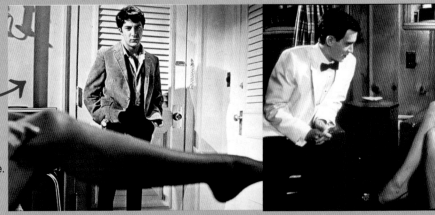

According to the experts at the American College of Sports Medicine, the average adult woman should aim for at least thirty minutes of cardio five times a week, plus two sessions of strength training. That may sound like a tall order, and for many of us, it is. (Lack of free time is probably the number one reason most mothers claim they can't or don't exercise.) Compounding matters is the fact that we are constantly bombarded by new workout fads, gadgets, and gear that promise to shave inches off our thighs, flatten our tummies, and give us tight, lifted butts that look as if they just stepped off the beaches of Rio. We convince ourselves that we just don't have time to work out or that without a certain piece of equipment or access to a certain gym, any amount of effort isn't worth the trouble. But the truth is that it shouldn't take mountains of equipment or an expensive gym membership to get a better body (not to mention the other benefits like a healthier heart, lower cholesterol, a lower risk of age-related diseases like osteoporosis, and the possibility of catching your son at tag once in a while).

Whether you've got a toddler (or two) balanced on your hip, or your kids are already in secondary school and you want to start working out again in earnest, this chapter aims to cut through the hype. It's not about some prescribed plan to lose XX amount of pounds in XX amount of weeks, nor is it about squeezing into a bathing suit by some arbitrary, insane deadline (like a month after delivery). According to celebrity trainer Ramona Braganza, who has worked with hard-bodies like Alba and Halle Berry, that shouldn't be the focus: "It's definitely about getting back to your healthy self, but taking your time and doing it right." Sounds like good advice to me.

1999 Comedic actress Jennifer Coolidge stars as sultry Stifler's mom (and has an affair with an eighteen-year-old high school senior) in the raucous *American Pie*.

2003 Sarah Jessica Parker shows off her flat stomach just six weeks after the birth of her son, James Wilkie Broderick, on the May cover of *W* magazine.

2003 Fountains of Wayne release their Grammy-nominated hit "Stacy's Mom," revolving around a young boy's fantasies about his girlfriend's mother. Real mom Rachel Hunter stars in the video.

2004 Mary-Louise Parker wins a Golden Globe just eighteen days after giving birth to her first child, William Atticus, and thanks him on the podium for making her "boobs look so good in this dress."

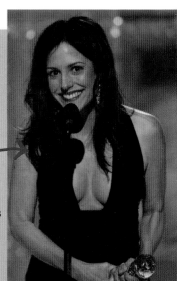

True or False: Common Diet Myths

Gossip Girl's Kelly Rutherford swears that she got her svelte shape just "running around after my kids," while Kourtney Kardashian says she dropped more than thirty pounds after her son Mason's birth by wearing something called a "Belly Bandit." Could these stories possibly be true? I would never categorically discount that there are things that work for some people and not others, and certainly we are not all built the same. However, most celebrity fitness pros think you shouldn't believe everything you read. Here's the scoop on what's fact and what's fiction.

You can get your body back just by "chasing after the children."

FALSE Although it's a myth perpetuated by countless celeb moms (and *may* be true for women who have already won the genetic lottery), staying two steps behind an active toddler is hardly the secret to a size 0. And while it's true that putting an exact number on how many calories you'll burn running alongside the kiddos is tough, let's be honest—it's not like you're training for a marathon. "New moms may burn a few extra calories, but probably not enough to actually lose much weight," says Jerry Mayo, Ph.D., an exercise physiologist and director of the Human Performance Lab at Arkansas Tech University. Still, every little bit helps,

...MORE HOT MOM PHENOM

2008 A bikini-clad Elisabeth Hasselback poses on the June cover of *Fitness* a mere seven weeks after delivering her second child.

2008 Jennifer Lopez completes the Malibu triathlon for charity on September 14, six months after having twins.

2009 *Cougar Town* premieres on ABC. A then-forty-five-year-old Courteney Cox had no trouble filming bikini scenes.

2009 Heidi Klum walks the Victoria's Secret runway less than six weeks after giving birth to her fourth child.

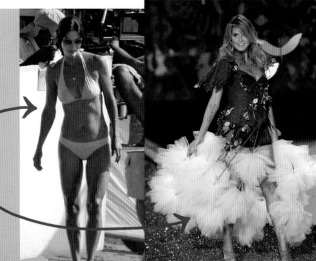

and chasing after your children is certainly better than spending an afternoon on the couch.

Drinking coffee before a workout helps you burn more calories.

TRUE Research has consistently shown that caffeine improves performance in endurance-type activities like running or cycling by making you feel more energized. Go ahead and have that mug of French roast before your morning workout; it may help you work out harder and longer and thus torch more calories.

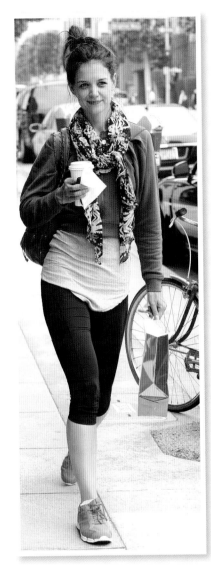

Katie Holmes

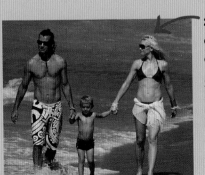

2011 Mom of two Gwen Stefani displays her awe-inspiring abs while on vacation in St. Bart's.

2011 Supermodel Miranda Kerr gets back to work for Victoria's Secret just three months after the birth of her first son, Flynn.

2011 Beyoncé announces that she's pregnant with her first child at the 2011 MTV Video Music Awards.

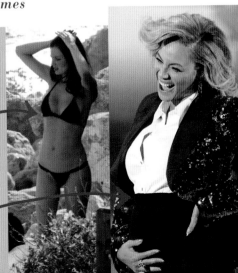

Wrapping or cinching your belly after giving birth will snap it back into shape.

FALSE (and sort of ridiculous). If squeezing into a girdlelike garment actually helped anybody lose weight, we'd all own a pair of Spanx and have tummies as toned as Gisele Bündchen's. Certified personal trainer Jessica Matthews, M.S., a member of the American Council on Exercise (ACE) agrees: "There is no solid evidence to support the notion that compression-style clothing aids in the process of losing weight or toning an area of the body." Spot reduction, by the way, or the idea that you can lose weight from just one specific area of the body (like the tummy), is also a myth.

What compression garments such as the Belly Bandit (worn by Hollywood moms like Bethenny Frankel and Minnie Driver) and the Tauts belly wrap (sold by celeb mom of four Brooke Burke) *may* do is help you fit more comfortably into your clothes, thereby providing a bit of a placebo effect. "You might feel more confident while wearing such a product," adds Matthews. "In turn, that may encourage you to exercise more intensely and frequently."

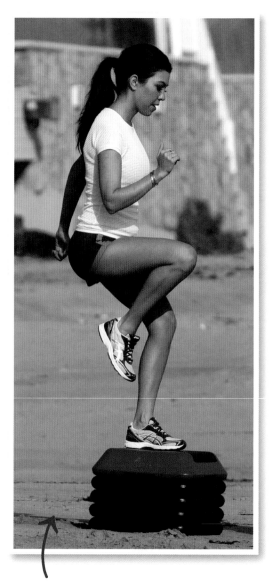

Exercise probably helped Kourtney Kardashian slim down more than the Belly Bandit.

Slim down before lifting weights or you'll build muscle over fat.

FALSE "You're going to get the fastest fat-burning results by lifting weights," says trainer Valerie Waters. So don't put it off. If you're still shedding the postpartum pounds, however, you will want to make sure you're getting plenty of cardio (to burn calories) and staying strict about your diet. If you watch what you eat, the body fat will come off and you'll be left with lean, sexy muscle.

Sleeping late can help you lose weight.

TRUE As every mom knows, sleep is a precious commodity. So when you're faced with the option of hitting the snooze button or getting up early to squeeze in a morning workout, which is the better bet? "If you're sleep-deprived," advises Dr. Mayo, "go ahead and skip the workout." According to recent research, women who sleep less than seven hours a night face an increased risk of weight gain and obesity. (If you're still in the throes of late-night feedings, regular naps can help bridge the gap.) Getting some rest and going into your next session

fresh allows for a better-quality workout anyway. Going to bed early, whenever possible, can also help you catch up on your beauty sleep. (Sometimes I actually go to bed at nine thirty P.M. It feels sort of geriatric . . . but also *great*!)

Lifting heavy weights will add bulk to your figure.

FALSE Women have very low levels of testosterone—the dominant male sex hormone, as well as the hormone needed to build big muscles—so even if you suddenly take up power-lifting, you're not going to turn into a female bodybuilder. (Think about it: Men are filled with testosterone, and even they sometimes have difficulty adding bulk.) Big, masculine-looking muscles also require loads of calories, lots of lean protein, and hours and hours in the gym. The main culprit in the battle of the bulge is food—protein shakes and bars loaded with calories and sugar, the bread basket at dinner, plus desserts, sodas, and processed snacks. Recent research confirms that lifting heavy weights, on the other hand, can help build strong bones and lean muscle and burn fat.

If you naturally have a very muscular

build, however, you may want to modify your moves. Waters suggests making an exercise more difficult as your strength improves, rather than picking up a heavier set of weights. "Change up the reps or shorten the amount of time you're resting between sets," she says. "There are so many different ways you can mix it up."

"But I Just Don't Have Time to Work Out!" and Other Roadblocks That Keep Us Overweight

I could probably come up with a million reasons—some with actual merit—why I don't have time to work out or why I just can't make it to the gym. For starters, I live in Los Angeles, so I'm always in my car. Whereas I used to be able to walk to work (or walk back home) while living in New York, in L.A. I am practically an invalid. No one walks anywhere here! I once had lunch with a colleague who picked the restaurant. We got in the car and drove... a whole three blocks. What I wouldn't give to be able to walk instead of drive my thirty-minute commute. These days, I hardly move my body at all, unless I make a real point of it.

Working out also requires some negotiation with my husband. If I want to go for a run in the morning, someone needs to make breakfast for the kids. And then, of course, I have that nagging mom guilt, feeling that where I should *really* be is at home with my children (not pounding the pavement in my running shoes). On the occasions that I actually get some exercise in before work, I'm busy wondering if my husband put the right grapes in the lunch boxes. (All this even though the world has never actually stopped while I put in thirty minutes on the elliptical at the Y.) Someone once told me that once you have kids, you'll never spend a free moment not worrying about *something*. It's so true.

Despite all those excuses, however, I can say—without hesitation—that no matter how badly I didn't want to get a workout in, I've never once regretted it afterward. I always feel a hundred times better after sweating out some of the stress and burning off some calories. Sometimes we just need a little help getting started. Here are some of the most common roadblocks in the path to getting fit and some advice on what you can do to get out of your own way.

PROBLEM

I have no time to work out. Seriously.

First of all, I know that women aren't exaggerating when they say they don't have much (or any) free time. But the reality is that being "too busy" to work out just isn't a valid excuse. It's up to you—and no one else—to make health and fitness a personal priority. And the notion that you have to spend hours and hours in the gym to lose the baby weight isn't true, anyway. In fact, personal trainer Mike Heatlie, who counts the supertoned Gwen Stefani as one of his celebrity clients, says that you should *never* train for more than one hour at a time, regardless of your schedule. If you're one of those moms who can't spare a whole hour all at once (and there are plenty of us who can't), you can still get results by breaking up your fitness regimen in intervals throughout the day.

As for what to do with that hour (or those stolen fifteen-minute intervals), most workout pros recommend circuit training—moving from one calisthenic exercise to the next with very little rest in between. "It's the most effective way to exercise, because circuit training works your entire body," says Waters. "You'll get a cardiovascular benefit, thanks to how hard you're working, as well as the benefits of strength training—shaping and toning of the muscles, plus the afterburn effect. Your metabolism will stay elevated, and you'll continue to burn calories even after your workout is over."

Many gyms offer classes that follow the circuit training philosophy (class descriptions should say so), while many personal trainers specialize in this type of workout. If you're unable or unwilling to hit the gym, however, it is possible to circuit train from home—a great option for evening workouts, since most of us are held hostage there after the kids go to bed. Try Waters's total body strength training workout (see next page); you can do it anywhere, and all you'll need is a soft ball and a resistance band with handles. Waters suggests doing the routine three times through, moving quickly from one exercise to the next, a minimum of three times a week. Even if you're a total exercise newbie or you're easing back into a workout routine, these eight basic moves are a fantastic starting point. Try them the next time you're watching reruns of *Top Chef* or giggling over *The Bachelor*. Instead of sprawling on the sofa, get up and get moving.

EXERCISE 1

The Glute Bridge with Ball

Lie on your back with both arms at your sides and your feet flat on the floor. Place a soft, squishy ball—a Swiss ball, an SPRI sponge ball, or even your child's plastic beach ball—between your knees. On an exhale, squeeze your bum and lift your hips until your body forms one straight line from head to knees, maintaining a gentle squeeze on the ball. Inhale as you lower your body back to the floor. Aim for 15 reps.

WORKS: *the butt and inner thighs.*

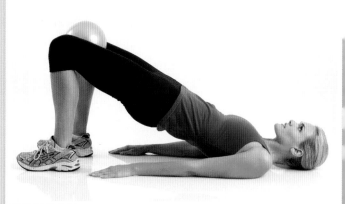

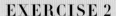

EXERCISE 2

The Plank

Lie on your stomach and get into a plank or push-up position, resting on your forearms and your toes. Suck in your abdominal muscles and keep your back and neck in a straight line. Hold for 30 to 60 seconds.

WORKS: *the entire core (otherwise known as the muscles in your pelvis, lower back, hips, and abdomen).*

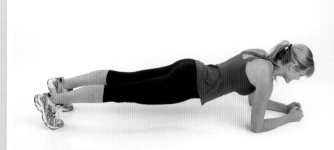

EXERCISE 3

The Side Plank

From the plank position, pivot to your side so the legs are stacked on top of each other and the feet are flexed, with your elbow resting on the floor directly under your shoulder. Place the opposite hand on your hip and raise the hips off the ground. Hold for 20 seconds. Then switch sides.

WORKS: *the entire core, especially the obliques (aka the "love handles").*

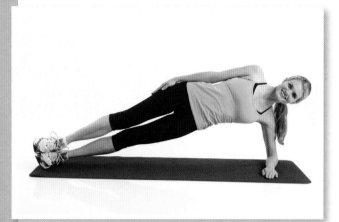

EXERCISE 4

The Standing Y

Start by standing with the feet hip-width apart, abs sucked in, and knees slightly bent. Then, bending at the waist, lean your torso forward at a forty-five-degree angle. Keeping your back flat, hang your arms straight down with your palms facing each other. While staying bent in the forty-five-degree angle, lift your arms up until they're at ear level, making sure that you're squeezing your arms up rather than using momentum to throw them up. In this position, your hands and arms will form the top of the "Y" and the rest of your body forms the base. Pause, then slowly return to the starting position. Aim for 10 reps.

WORKS: *the shoulders, upper and lower back.*

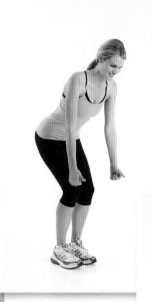

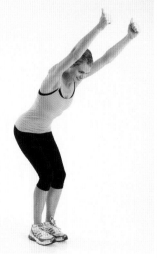

EXERCISE 5

The Standing T

Again, start by standing with the feet hip-width apart, abs sucked in, and knees slightly bent. Then, bending at the waist, lean your torso forward at a forty-five-degree angle. Keeping your back flat, hang your arms straight down with the thumbs turned out. Now, raise your arms straight out to the side (with your thumbs facing toward the ceiling), until the arms are perpendicular to your body, forming a "T." At the top range of the motion, squeeze your shoulder blades together. Pause, then slowly return to the starting position. Aim for 10 reps.

WORKS: *the backs of the shoulders and the midback.*

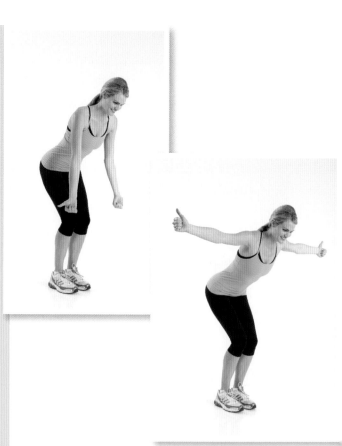

EXERCISE 6

The Incline Push-up

Get into a push-up position on an elevated surface (like a bench or a step, so your hands are on the step and your feet are on the floor). Lower yourself until your chest is two inches from the surface and then push back up, making sure that your head remains in a neutral position by looking straight ahead. If this exercise is too difficult, you can do the push-ups on your knees. Aim for 8 to 10 reps.

WORKS: *the chest, shoulders, and triceps.*

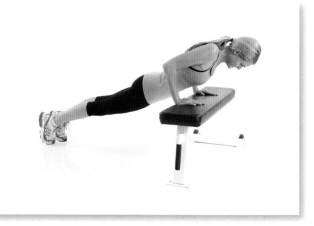

EXERCISE 7

The Squat and Row

For this exercise, you'll need a resistance band with handles (Waters recommends the bands from performbetter.com, but you can find resistance bands in any sporting goods store). Start by anchoring the band around a heavy object, or use the door attachment that comes with most models. Then, holding the handles with your arms extended in front of you, squat down slowly, pulling your elbows back and squeezing your shoulder blades together, as if you were rowing a boat. Aim for 12 to 15 reps.

WORKS: *the midback, thighs, butt, core.*

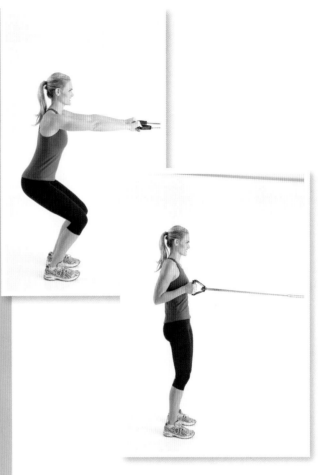

EXERCISE 8

The Dip

Sit on the edge of a bench or a chair, gripping it with both hands, feet placed firmly on the ground. Push yourself up (using your triceps) until your arms are straight, and then lower yourself back down so that your elbows are at a ninety-degree angle. Keep your bum close to the edge of the chair while performing the exercise, and don't scrunch your shoulders—push up through them. Aim for 10 to 12 reps.

WORKS: *the triceps and shoulders.*

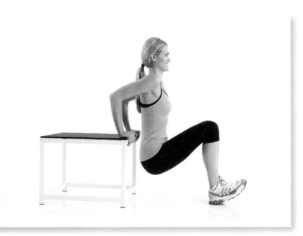

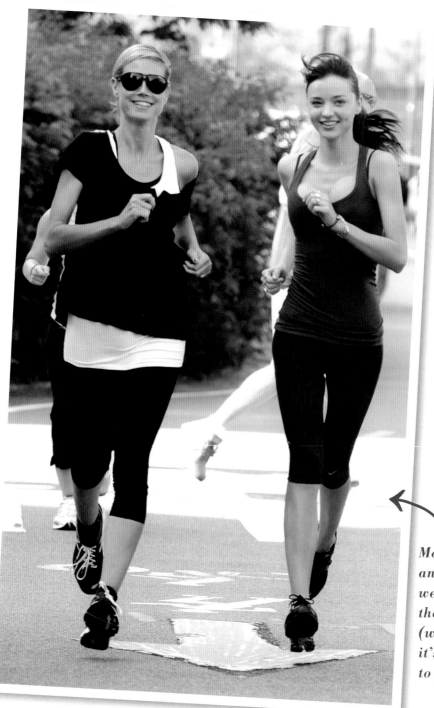

Moms Heidi Klum and Miranda Kerr were fit before they got pregnant (which helps), but it's never too late to get in shape!

PROBLEM

I'm pregnant and don't feel like waddling around the gym.

When you're expecting, you may feel like devouring a sleeve of Oreos, taking a three-hour afternoon nap, or—thanks to raging hormones—telling your husband where he can stick it; working out probably isn't at the top of your to-do list. Regular exercise is not only vital to the health of your baby, it will likely make the delivery process (as well as the struggle to lose the baby weight) so much easier. Unfortunately, about one out of every five American women is already obese by the time she becomes pregnant, according to researchers at the Centers for Disease Control. And that obesity can cause all sorts of problems—in addition to record high rates of C-sections, overweight moms-to-be are more likely to suffer complications like gestational diabetes, hemorrhage, blood clots, and strokes during pregnancy and childbirth. Studies also show that babies born to obese women are nearly three times as likely to die within three months of delivery; obese women are about twice as likely to have a stillbirth. (I don't mean to scare you, but it's true.)

Even if you're at a normal, healthy weight, there are plenty of reasons to make exercise a priority—nearly every fitness pro will tell you that staying fit both before and during pregnancy will help you bounce back that much faster. "Getting into shape doesn't start after the baby comes out," adds New York City–based personal trainer David Kirsch, who's helped Heidi Klum and Liv Tyler regain their pre-baby bodies. "It's about your level of fitness *before* pregnancy."

Of course, you will want to modify your workout routine so as not to raise your heart rate *too* much (ask your doctor about that old recommendation of maxing out at 140 beats per minute; many now say going higher may be fine if you are already fit). Trade high-impact moves for low-impact activities like walking or swimming. "Power walking outside is amazing," says Kirsch. "Or try walking on a treadmill at an incline; anywhere from 3 to 5 percent is great." If you're still too self-conscious to hit the gym (or walk outside), look for an at-home workout DVD that's tailored to pregnant women.

stop! before you eat *that*, consider this...

Admit it. That sign posted at your favorite chain restaurant alerting you to the number of calories that are really in that minimuffin has made you rethink your food choices (or at least made you feel guiltier about them). And that's just the point. Who needs to start the day with 490 calories from a slice of banana-nut loaf? Not you. Los Angeles–based nutritionist and weight loss expert Christine Avanti, the woman responsible for the sleek physiques of Chelsea Handler and celeb mom Samantha Harris (and creator of the nutritional resource christineavanti.com), breaks down the cost of those high-calorie foods. Makes you seriously question if that slice of pizza or chocolate cake is really worth the subsequent sweat session!

Food	Calories/ Grams Fat	Exercise Needed
Oversize vanilla cupcake with chocolate frosting	475; 24 g	1 hour running
Snack-size bag of Doritos	250; 13 g	1.25 hours walking the dog
5-ounce glass of Champagne	100; 0 g	1 hour cooking
Quarter-pound cheeseburger	408; 16 g	1 hour tennis
Medium French fries	380; 19 g	1 hour walking up a hill
Standard hot dog	377; 15 g	1 hour race walking
8-ounce frozen margarita	445; 0 g	2.5 hours surfing
Slice of pepperoni pizza	324; 13 g	1 hour ballroom dancing
Small ice-cream sundae	279; 7 g	1.25 hours yoga

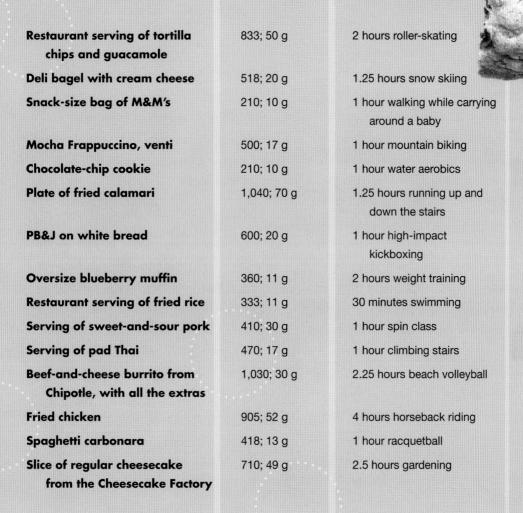

Restaurant serving of tortilla chips and guacamole	833; 50 g	2 hours roller-skating
Deli bagel with cream cheese	518; 20 g	1.25 hours snow skiing
Snack-size bag of M&M's	210; 10 g	1 hour walking while carrying around a baby
Mocha Frappuccino, venti	500; 17 g	1 hour mountain biking
Chocolate-chip cookie	210; 10 g	1 hour water aerobics
Plate of fried calamari	1,040; 70 g	1.25 hours running up and down the stairs
PB&J on white bread	600; 20 g	1 hour high-impact kickboxing
Oversize blueberry muffin	360; 11 g	2 hours weight training
Restaurant serving of fried rice	333; 11 g	30 minutes swimming
Serving of sweet-and-sour pork	410; 30 g	1 hour spin class
Serving of pad Thai	470; 17 g	1 hour climbing stairs
Beef-and-cheese burrito from Chipotle, with all the extras	1,030; 30 g	2.25 hours beach volleyball
Fried chicken	905; 52 g	4 hours horseback riding
Spaghetti carbonara	418; 13 g	1 hour racquetball
Slice of regular cheesecake from the Cheesecake Factory	710; 49 g	2.5 hours gardening

PROBLEM
I've just given birth, and don't know how long to wait before working out.

Not so long ago, nearly all new moms were advised to wait six whole weeks before embarking on a postdelivery workout routine. These days, however, it's generally considered safe to start exercising right away, provided you had an uncomplicated vaginal birth. But even if you're eager to break a sweat—and you've gotten a green light from your doctor—it's important to take it slow: "If there's too much focus on 'I've got to get my body back' too soon, you could wind up with a long-term injury," warns Heatlie. For quick—but safe—results, he takes celeb clients through a three-part process:

1. Recovery
Though some new mothers may be raring to go, women who have had a C-section or a complicated birth may take a little longer to get back in the exercise saddle. For the first four to six weeks after delivery, try focusing on low-impact pelvic floor exercises (or Kegels) and core conditioning moves (you can read more about these on the next page). "All of those internal stomach muscles have been seriously weakened by pregnancy and childbirth, and they need to be strengthened," says Heatlie. You can also ease back into a cardio routine by walking or swimming a few times a week.

2. Conditioning
Around six weeks postdelivery, you can slowly start to ramp up your routine by melding higher-impact exercises (like jumping jacks, jumping rope, running, and some step aerobics) with light to moderate weight training.

3. Ab Blasting
By twelve weeks, you should be able to train at your highest intensity—so now's the time to focus on losing the belly fat as well as toning your hips, butt, and arms. "With hard work, good diet, and consistent training, you can actually get your body looking even better than it did before baby," says Heatlie.

PROBLEM
I can't ditch my mom pooch!

While certain exercises can remedy a post-baby paunch, you'll actually want to avoid traditional crunches. "Crunches won't help because they're not activating your deep core muscles," says Cynthia M. Chiarello, P.T., Ph.D., assistant professor of clinical physical therapy at Columbia University. Celebrity personal trainers agree. "I once helped a client take five inches off her waist in five weeks, just by stopping her from doing sit-ups and having her switch to more core conditioning work," says Heatlie.

So what exercises *will* help you whittle your waistline? Moves that target the transverse abdominis, the sheet of muscle that lies directly underneath your would-be six-pack (this section of muscle wraps around your midsection like a belt; so the tighter it is, the tinier your waist will be).

The plank and the side plank are two such exercises, as is the abdominal vacuum, which you can perform from a seated position by exhaling all the air from your lungs, then using your belly muscles to suck in your stomach, as if you were pulling your belly button back to your spine. Hold, then release. Pelvic floor exercises, or Kegels, can also help tighten up the core.

Still can't seem to trim the tummy? Sometimes a post-baby paunch is just fat, says Dr. Chiarello. And if that's the case, it's time to take a closer look at your diet—extra calories could be contributing to the problem.

3 exercises to do in the car

Most busy moms spend an insane amount of time driving from one end of town to the other. Next time you strap on your seat belt, remember: The abdominal vacuum, glute squeezes, and Kegel exercises can be performed (safely!) from the comfort of the driver's seat. It's kind of nice to know that you can start tightening your core—even when you're stuck waiting for school to let out.

1. The abdominal vaccuum Exhale all the air from your lungs, then use your ab muscles to suck in your stomach, as if you were pulling your belly button back to your spine. Hold, then release. Shoot for 3 reps of 10 seconds each.

2. The Kegel To do a Kegel, tighten and release the pelvic muscles—the same muscles that you would use to stop the flow of urine. Work up to 3 sets of 10.

3. The glute squeeze Kelly Ripa once admitted to doing these in her car. The concept is pretty simple: Tighten your stomach muscles and squeeze your glutes. Hold, then release. Try for 10 reps.

PROBLEM

I feel guilty even thinking about getting a personal trainer.

Lots of new moms probably think that enlisting the help of a personal trainer is something only a wealthy A-list actress would do, akin to hiring a personal chef or traveling the world with a professional hair and makeup team (if only!). But the truth is that hiring professional help can have potentially huge benefits, and it doesn't have to cost a fortune.

For one thing, a qualified trainer will tailor workouts to your specific needs, so you can reap the maximum rewards from your thirty- or sixty-minute session—that's a big advantage if you're strapped for time. Accountability, of course, is another benefit. "I don't think a group exercise instructor or a DVD is going to call and ask why you didn't show up for a workout," says Dr. Mayo. "If you're going to pay for it, you're probably more likely to go, and that's half the battle." A trainer also can make sure you're not doing too much too soon after delivery (one reason that Heatlie suggests enlisting a trainer soon after birth), as well as determine when you need to be pushed and in what capacity. After all, a halfhearted effort on the elliptical probably isn't going to get you bikini-ready. (You can ask trainers if they are schooled in training postnatal women; there is such a thing as a postnatal certification.) Finally, a trainer can ensure that you're performing those all-important core conditioning moves, like Kegels and the plank, correctly. "The transverse abdominis is a very deep muscle and therefore difficult to target," says Dr. Chiarello.

If a personal trainer seems way outside your price range, consider this: Though prices may range from as low as $30 an hour to as high as $300 an hour, depending on the experience of the trainer and your geographic location, many gyms offer a free orientation when you join. You can also try signing up for just a few sessions—rather than making a long-term commitment—then checking back in with your pro periodically to make sure you're still on track. Most trainers will write down a program for you to follow all on your own. To find a local personal trainer who has been certified by the American Council on Exercise, visit acefitness.org.

PROBLEM

I'm too embarrassed to work out in front of other people.

There's a simple solution here: Buy a workout DVD from an established trainer or fitness facility. Fitness DVDs have come a *lonnng* way since the cheesy aerobics videos of the 1980s; they're often just as intense as any class offered at your local gym and, of course, you can do them from the comfort of your own home. Try one of these celeb mom favorites:

Aerobarre

Victoria's Secret supermodel Adriana Lima, who—perhaps not surprisingly—managed to drop her baby weight in a matter of months, is a fan of this unique fifty-minute combination ballet, boxing, and sculpting workout. Expect a high-energy routine set to hard-driving beats, with instructions easy enough for anyone to follow. Devotees will notice sleeker arms and legs and a trimmer core. ($20; aerospacenyc.com)

Ramona Braganza's 321 Baby Bulge Be Gone

The combo of cardio, circuit training, and core exercises worked for Jessica Alba and Halle Berry, and chances are you'll see improvements, too. Build up your endurance and strength through three post-baby workout phases in this three-DVD program. Follow the nutritional guidelines (included), and celeb trainer Braganza swears you can shave off as many as twenty to twenty-five pounds in three months. ($30 each or $75 for all three DVDs; ramonabraganza.com)

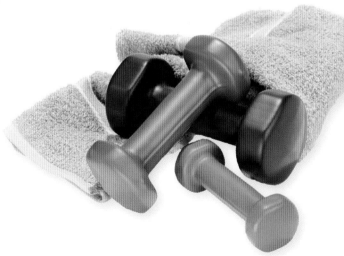

P90X

"I like that it has a little bit of everything," busy mom Sheryl Crow has said of this twelve-DVD set, which includes workouts focused on the legs and back, shoulders and arms, and, of course, the abs. The mix of high-intensity routines will keep boredom at bay while burning calories at maximum capacity. Poppy Montgomery swears that P90X helped her drop seventy pounds of baby weight! ($120; beachbody.com)

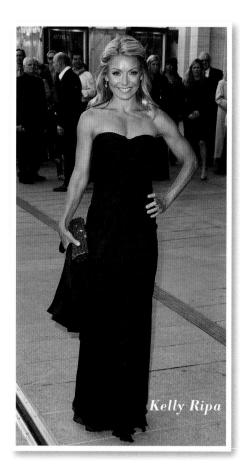

Kelly Ripa

Sheryl Crow

Physique 57 Classic 57 Minute Full Body Workout

Mom of three Kelly Ripa calls this New York ballet barre class "the love of my life... besides my husband." The just-shy-of-an-hour workout melds intervals of isometric exercises (think squat pulses and leg lifts) with core work and deep stretches. ($25; physique57.com)

Pilates Weight Loss for Beginners

If your eyes glaze over at the mere mention of "the roll-up" or "standing saw," let Brooke Siler, who's trained Rachel Weisz and Madonna, take you through the basics of Pilates in this fifty-minute mat-and-cardio routine. The best part? There are modifications for most exercises, making the program accessible to anyone at any level. ($10; amazon.com)

YogaWorks Body Slim

Moms like Kate Hudson and Sarah Jessica Parker get long and lean with sun salutations at YogaWorks' NYC and L.A. studios. You can get the same sculpting and calorie-burning benefits with this vigorous fifty-minute series of yoga poses. ($11; yogaworks.com)

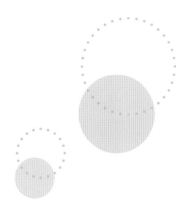

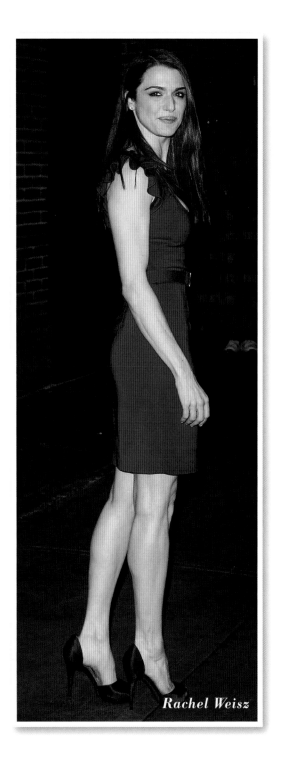

Rachel Weisz

PROBLEM

I lost a few pounds, but now I'm stuck.

One thing you definitely don't want to do is stay within your comfort zone for too long—falling into a scripted pattern at the gym will only trigger a plateau in your weight loss. "Our bodies adapt very quickly, so a move that initially burned fifty calories might only burn twenty-five after several weeks of workouts," says Waters. "Mixing things up ensures that you'll keep getting results. It also keeps you mentally fresh—you'll get bored if you just do the same thing over and over." For optimum results, she suggests switching up your routine at least every six weeks.

If you want to know whether or not you're working out *hard* enough (or perhaps even too hard), consider investing in a heart rate monitor. "These are great motivational tools because—by comparing one workout to the next—you can compete against *yourself*," says Braganza, who uses the device with celebrity clients including Jessica Alba and Halle Berry. What a heart rate monitor *won't* do, however, is tell you your target "fat-burning zone." "This is a myth," says Dr. Mayo. "When it comes to weight loss, the key is to burn more calories. More than anything, heart rate zones are used for exercise safety." While there are plenty of online calculators available to determine your target heart rate, it's best to consult a physician, especially if you're pregnant.

In terms of your expectations, you should aim for losing no more than two pounds a week, keeping in mind that the first five pounds might fall off much faster than the last five. If after six months you're still not getting the results you want, despite working out regularly and watching your diet, consult your doctor. You could have a thyroid condition or a hormonal imbalance (or even food allergies) that may be preventing weight loss.

PROBLEM

I have zero motivation.

Too often, I've found that my motivation to hit the gym comes only when there is an immediate goal at hand, like I have to wear a tight dress to an event...*tomorrow.* Recently, I had the brilliant idea to call up my long-lost trainer to work out my arms—the morning before I had to wear a strapless dress. (Better late than never?) Clearly, the list of things I'd rather do than hit the gym is long and varied, but once I've gotten into a groove, working out becomes (once again) an essential part of my life, kind of like brushing my teeth.

We all need some strategies to light that workout fire. Personal trainer Jessica Matthews suggests that a mix of extrinsic rewards (like indulging in that deep-tissue massage or purchasing that slim-fitting bandage dress) and intrinsic strategies (like the sense of accomplishment you'll feel at the end of an intense yoga class) is your surest bet for long-term success. Try some of these tried-and-true tactics to keep you committed:

Invest in an iPod or some other MP3 player Studies have shown that listening to music can motivate you to exercise longer and harder (there's a reason they don't blast NPR on the stereo at the gym). So buy that iPod or MP3 player and load it with songs that will really get you moving, whether that's today's chart toppers or hits from the 1970s and 1980s. "Songs that have meaning to you will give you an adrenaline boost so you can really lose yourself in the workout," says Michael Olajide Jr., trainer to Adriana Lima and co-owner of boxing gym Aerospace NYC. "Ultimately, you'll associate a positive experience with sweating and making your muscles burn."

Use the buddy system This one's obvious—by enlisting a friend to work out with you, you'll be less likely to cancel your training session at the last minute. After all, your girlfriend won't be so forgiving if you stand her up at spinning class three days in a row. Plus, research shows that women (and men) who have a support network of encouraging friends and family are more likely to reach their weight loss goals than those who go it alone. If you have a workout buddy (or buddies), consider purchasing group sessions with a trainer. The small group approach can enhance motivation while also cutting down on the cost.

Recruit your husband Spending day after day cooped up with tiny tots—especially if you're a stay-at-home mom—can make any woman crave a little "me time," so strike a deal with your husband. Have him watch the kiddos for an hour in the evening (even if it's after they've already gone to sleep) so you can have an hour all to yourself. Equating the gym (or the yoga studio or the running trails in the park) with a reprieve from mommy duty can make even the least motivated among us practically desperate to feel the burn.

Shoot for just 10 minutes You could do practically anything for ten minutes, right? Of course you could. So plan to speed walk on the treadmill or pop in that Pilates DVD for ten minutes only. If that turns out to be all you can manage, fine. Chances are, however, that once you've completed those ten minutes, you're going to keep going. "We have a saying at the gym: Energy begets energy," says Olajide Jr. "If you give energy, you will receive energy." Sometimes a little push is all it takes to get going.

Set attainable goals Setting multiple-range goals can also help keep you motivated. For example, Matthews suggests establishing a short-term or weekly goal (like, "I will work out three days this week"), a medium-term or monthly goal ("I will lose five pounds by the end of this month") and a long-term goal, somewhere around the six-month mark ("I will be wearing my pre-pregnancy clothes by August"). Be sure to continually evaluate and adjust your goals to ensure continued progress and success.

how many calories do those workouts burn?

Some forms of exercise, like Pilates and yoga, may burn fewer calories but provide benefits like increased flexibility and core strength.*

Barre class	300 calories
Biking outside (moderate intensity)	514 calories
Boot camp class	548 calories
Boxing	579 calories
Circuit training	514 calories
Cross-country skiing (moderate intensity)	514 calories
Dance cardio	309 calories
Downhill skiing (moderate intensity)	386 calories
Elliptical machine (moderate intensity)	418 calories
Hiking, cross-country	386 calories
Horseback riding	257 calories
Kickboxing	643 calories
Pilates (beginner)	225 calories
Race walking	418 calories
Running (10-minute-mile pace)	643 calories
Snowboarding (moderate intensity)	386 calories
Snowshoeing	450 calories
Spinning class (moderate intensity)	707 calories
Stair-climbing	579 calories
Stationary bike	450 calories
Swimming (moderate intensity)	450 calories
Tai chi	257 calories
Tennis (singles)	514 calories
Walking (moderate intensity)	212 calories
Weight lifting (moderate intensity)	193 calories
Yoga (low intensity, like Iyengar)	161 calories
Yoga (high intensity, like a flow class)	431 calories

*Calories based on a 135-pound woman working out for 1 hour.

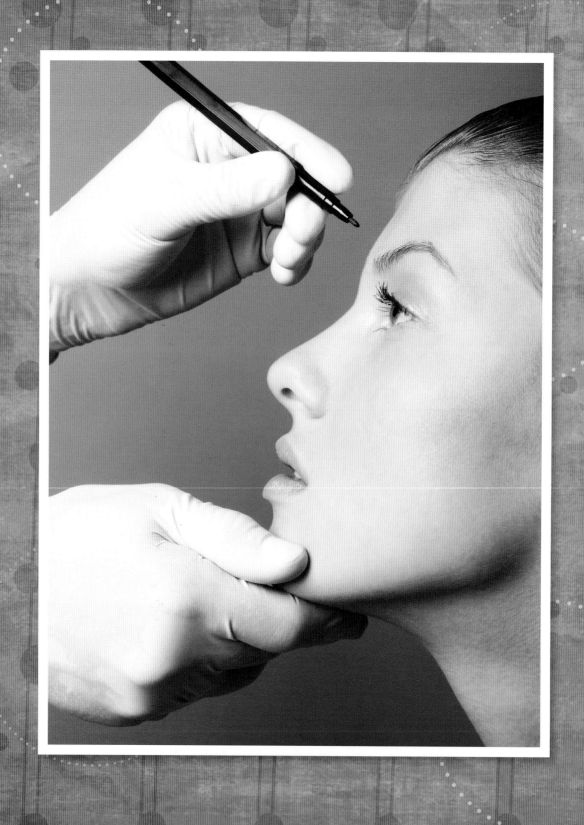

do your boobs hang low?

How to Know If Botox or Plastic Surgery Is for You

I have lived in two cities—New York and Los Angeles—where there is a preponderance of noticeably older dads: dads with gray hair, dads who look like they could be grandpas, dads who are on their second (sometimes third) families, dads with paunchy guts and double chins (and I'm assuming a lot of money). But the moms? In these image-obsessed coastal cities, the mothers look pretty fantastic. Very, very few of them have gray hair—one of my sons recently asked my husband why he is so gray compared to me (ha!)—the clothes are usually on trend (after all, these cities set the shopping standard for the rest of the country), and the kind of obesity that afflicts much of middle America is just not that prevalent. On the contrary, moms in New York and L.A. look more like they subsist purely on lettuce leaves. Have you ever seen any of the satirical websites that "make over" celebrities as if they lived in

Ohio or Wisconsin? (Some of the most glamorous stars are Photoshopped with frizzy hair and fat arms.) Admittedly, they're hilarious. But sites like these point to a painfully obvious truth: Women from the left and right coasts tend to spend more money on self-maintenance than anyone else in the country.

More recently, however, I've noticed the rise of a disturbing trend: something I'm going to call "Frankenmom."

These are the women who look like some kind of science experiment gone awry. Their ages—even the generation from which they hail—are not entirely clear, and their faces are some kind of Picasso-style abstract of huge lips, overarched eyebrows, and pinched little noses and cheekbones that have been sculpted by some doctor you'd swear was blind. And forget about the boobs. Here in L.A., the real Silicon Valley of America, women of all ages walk around in all manner of bursting-at-the-seams tank tops, as if they were vying for the last available job at Hooters. Recently, I was at a pool party for one of my son's young friends, and my husband and I had a very real and very legitimate (also very private) conversation about whether some of the mothers, based on the way they looked and dressed, had ever worked as professional escorts.

Discussing who has and who hasn't had plastic surgery is one of life's mindless parlor games; it's lame, it's cheap, it's even mean. But we all do it. Partly it stems from just pure unadulterated cattiness, the kind we hate to see in our children but of which we are sometimes guilty. Part of it is wishful thinking, the hope that a really beautiful woman *must* be getting work done (somehow, this evens out the balance sheet in our minds). And part of it is that deep-down temptation we all sometimes struggle with, the lingering thought that maybe we could or should get a little work done, too; so we mercilessly critique the faces of our friends and of famous people. I once had a woman over who *insisted* we go through the photos of one of her female friends on Facebook to determine whether or not she'd secretly been getting Botox. We probably blew thirty minutes on this endeavor…if only the poor woman knew about our silly adventure. (By the way, the verdict was yes. Big-time.)

Plastic surgeons have a different, less off-putting name for the growing Frankenmom phenomenon—it's called the "mommy makeover," or the packaging together of several surgical procedures, typically a breast augmentation, tummy tuck, and liposuction, to "reverse" the effects of childbirth. The message is more than a little disturbing. Women have been having babies since the dawn of humanity; do we really mean to imply that a sagging breast or a stomach pooch is so unnatural and so unsightly that it merits a surgical intervention? Yet more than 325,000 women underwent some sort of mommy makeover in 2006, according to the American Society of Plastic Surgeons. (Since "mommy makeover" is a marketing term and not a scientific one, statistics are hard to come by; but I'm sure the trend has only grown in popularity in the last few years.) The takeaway seems to be that even as the men in our lives age, gain weight, go bald, or get gray, and our children grow and mature with each passing year, women should remain somehow frozen in time, perpetually age thirty and "perfect." (Messed up, right?)

It is with some ambivalence, then, that I write this chapter. Personally, I have a number of problems with plastic surgery. It's almost exclusively for the wealthy (I actually think a lot of the unusually strange faces I see in L.A. are worn as badges of honor—it conveys *extreme* affluence); voluntary surgery that carries a risk of injury or death seems like a pretty bad idea when you have a child or two depending on you; and last, is it not kind of creepy and wrong? I mean, who is setting these

standards of "beauty" anyway and why do we all follow along? Having said that, however, I recognize that we all indulge in medical solutions to aesthetic problems, from having braces as a child to laser hair removal. So where on the continuum does it become too much? Surgery may be the only solution to correct, say, pounds of sagging skin left over from a multiples birth. I recognize, too, that a conservative amount of Botox doesn't have to look unnatural, nor does it necessarily make you a vain or superficial person. In fact, Botox, injectables, and laser treatments, all of which are classified as noninvasive and nonsurgical, may be more palatable for women who would like to look a little younger or a little more well rested without having to go under the knife (which, unless you want a full-on facelift, is not even common practice anymore). This chapter will go over the basics of what's out there and available, to help you determine if a cosmetic procedure is right for you. But please, don't turn yourself into a Frankenmom. Kids have enough nightmares to contend with.

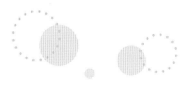

What a Dermatologist Can Do for You

BOTOX

So many celebrity moms have 'fessed up about their Botox use that it seems about as commonplace as getting a blowout or a teeth cleaning (at least in L.A.). Jenny McCarthy, Daisy Fuentes, and Jennie Garth have all spoken openly about going "under the needle." Actress Virginia Madsen even acts as a celebrity spokesperson for the manufacturer. Clearly, admitting to Botox use is no longer taboo. In fact, I have a growing number of friends who will casually mention that they just got shot up during their lunch break. It's perhaps no wonder,

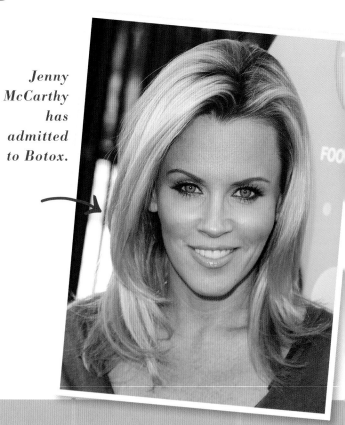

Jenny McCarthy has admitted to Botox.

warning!

Most doctors recommend that new mothers wait *at least* six months after delivery before undergoing any kind of elective surgical procedure; no procedure should even be considered while you're still breastfeeding. (No study has even been done to determine if Botox affects a mother's breast milk…but do you really want to be the first to find out?) Any surgery involving the abdominal area (like a tummy tuck) or the genitals (such as a labiaplasty) should be avoided entirely until you are finished bearing children. Many physicians also recommend that all prospective patients be in excellent health, eat a healthy diet, have a regular workout routine, and have lost the baby weight before going under the knife. Surgery is serious and should never be thought of as a "quick fix."

then, that injections of botulism toxin, a protein produced by a strain of bacteria that paralyzes muscles, have become the single most common cosmetic procedure in the country (5 million injections were performed in 2008), according to the American Society of Plastic Surgeons. Of course, Botox has noncosmetic uses, too: Years before California plastic surgeon Richard Clark figured out that it can iron out frown lines, the toxin was used to help people with cerebral palsy calm their muscle spasms and to paralyze overly tight muscles in people with crossed eyes. More recently, Botox has been used to treat migraines and hyperhidrosis (overactive sweat glands). By and large, however, Botox is used to flatten wrinkles, specifically those caused by the face's animation, like laughing, squinting, and frowning. So if you're bothered by deep creases along the forehead, the little "11" between your eyebrows that pops out whenever you frown, or crow's-feet at the corners of your eyes, Botox can help—for about three to six months. That's right, Botox isn't permanent, so you'll have to come in for repeat injections to maintain the desired effect.

In the wrong hands, Botox injections can cause temporary side effects (like a persistent headache or a drooping eyelid) or leave you with a sort of shocked deer-

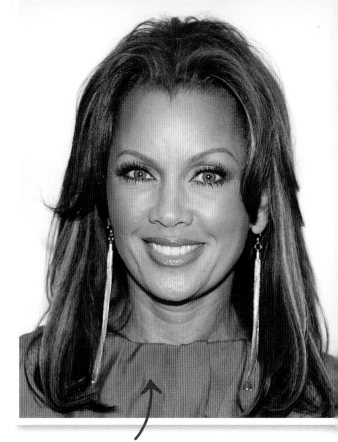

Wrinkle-free mom Vanessa Williams has said that she "loves" Botox.

in-headlights look or an overly immobile, flat forehead and face. (We've all seen celebrities who were once beautiful and now look, well, strange. Or take a look at the women on your local TV news—it's an epidemic there, too.) For that reason, it's imperative to select a qualified dermatologist or plastic surgeon to perform your injections. You do not want to get Botox from an aesthetician who spends most of her time giving facials or Brazilian waxes, or from someone who works out of the back room in your neighborhood nail salon. "You have to pick a doctor who has an artful eye," says New York dermatologist David Colbert. "He or she has to understand the bones, the nerves, the muscles. In other words, they have to have good taste. If you go to a female dermatologist and she can't move her face, for example, you might be in the wrong office." Remember: fewer lines = improvement. No lines = freakshow.

THE PROCESS Plan to allot about an hour for the appointment. In terms of pain, the injections aren't terribly comfortable, but, hey, you've experienced childbirth—you'll be fine. Since some minor bruising is possible, you might not want to schedule the injections immediately before an important work meeting or a big party. Full results may not be apparent until a week after treatment.

THE BILL Anywhere from $300 to $1,000 per treatment, depending on how much solution is being injected.

RESTYLANE AND JUVÉDERM

As we get older, one of the many joys we can look forward to is that our bones shrink even as our waistlines grow. Some of the sagging we may begin to see on our faces and necks as we head into our late thirties is caused in part by the shrinking of the bones in the face, as well as the gradual loss of volume in our cheeks, near the temples, and under the eyes. While Botox is used to paralyze muscles, facial *fillers* are used to fill in grooves and hollows in the face. In other words, fillers can "put back" what time takes away. And they are also ripe for abuse. That crazy fake cheekbone look that a number of aging actresses have? It's from having too much filler injected into their cheeks to prop up sagging skin with structural support. Again, moderation is best.

Restylane and Juvéderm are the pharmaceutical names for different brands of fillers made from synthetic hyaluronic acid, a key component of cell structure. Most commonly they are injected into the nasolabial folds that emanate from your nostrils down to your chin, those "marionette lines" or smile lines around the mouth, and sometimes the hollows under the eyes (to conceal dark circles), or they can be used to make the lips and cheekbones fuller and softer in appearance. Like Botox injections, fillers are pricey and they don't last forever; to maintain the results, you'll be returning to the doctor's office every five to nine months. Injections into the nasolabial folds may be more painful than Botox injections to the forehead, so you may want to ask your doctor for a dental block (the same anesthetic dentists administer before drilling away the decay of a cavity). Or talk to your doctor about using a filler that includes lidocaine (an anesthetic) as part of its formulation.

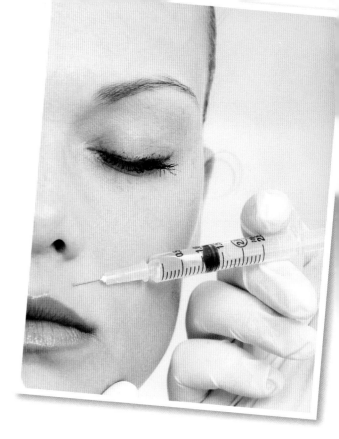

THE PROCESS As with Botox, you'll want to allot about an hour for the appointment. However, with fillers the results are instantaneous. Bruising, especially in the cheek area and under the eyes, is common, since the needles must penetrate deeper into the skin than the needles used in Botox injections.

THE BILL Typically a bit pricier than Botox; anywhere from $500 to $1,000 per treatment.

LASER RESURFACING

Laser treatments, of which there are many types, may be used for a variety of reasons: to smooth and soften wrinkles, to firm and tighten the skin, to boost collagen production, to remove brown spots and damage, or for permanent hair removal. They also can help the skin appear refreshed and "new." Personally, I love lasers—I've been a fan of the Fraxel laser for a few years now—and think they can actually deliver results, as opposed to expensive beauty products that rarely do.

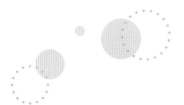

Intense Pulse Light (IPL)

Intense Pulse Light (IPL) treatments, sometimes called "photorejuvenation" or "photofacial" treatments, use a type of low-level laser to reduce hyperpigmentation, like age or liver spots, sun damage, melasma, redness associated with rosacea, and fine lines and wrinkles (when used over multiple sessions). IPL treatments also may help the pores appear smaller and may be a preventive measure against lines and wrinkles, especially when used by younger women. IPL treatments are also "nonablative," which means they don't damage the surface of the skin (unlike some chemical peels, which "peel" off the top layers of skin, leaving you oozing and raw). You may experience some minor redness immediately after IPL treatments, but that generally subsides within a few days.

Fraxel Certain kinds of lasers also may be used to treat striae distensae, otherwise known as stretch marks. The relatively new Fraxel laser, for example, uses pulses of light to zap only parts of the scar over the course of several treatments. The body responds by producing new collagen and epithelium, a type of animal tissue. (The epidermis, or skin, is a type of epithelium.) In a 2007 clinical trial, five to six treatments resulted in a 75 percent improvement of stretch marks, while a 2007 Brazilian clinical study showed that fractional laser resurfacing improved both the texture and the appearance of mature, white striae (older stretch marks that are silvery in appearance), though the procedure works best for lighter skin tones.

Fraxel can also be used to improve a whole raft of other skin woes: fine wrinkles (especially around the eyes), age spots and sun spots, acne scars, and, of course, melasma. I've had the procedure done several times to wipe away my melasma; for me, it has worked beautifully. And your skin looks pretty great for several months, as your face is building up collagen during the healing process. I know one doctor who claims that a few Fraxel sessions are the equivalent to wiping five years off your face. I'm not going to vouch for *that*, but I will say it does offer immediate improvement.

THE PROCESS Laser treatments are more intensive than Botox or filler injections and require a bit more advance planning. The treatment for Fraxel, in particular, typically begins with numbing cream placed on the area to be treated. The actual application of the laser is well under thirty minutes, during which time you'll be asked to wear tiny goggles (like the kind people wear inside tanning booths). Because Fraxel treatments aren't comfortable (imagine little hot needles being poked all over your face) some doctors' offices will offer patients Demerol, Xanax, or Vicodin (just be prepared to have someone drive you home). Regardless of whether you opt for IPL or Fraxel, you'll look as though you have a mild sunburn for a few days afterward; light peeling is also common for up to a week.

THE BILL IPL treatments average around $500 per session; Fraxel treatments can run between $1,000 and $1,500 for a single session.

SKIN TIGHTENING AND CELLULITE REDUCTION

Certain kinds of lasers—called "radio-frequency" lasers—also may be used to firm and tighten the skin or to reduce cellulite, the cottage cheese–like dimpling you might sometimes see on your thighs or bum. These lasers work by stimulating the growth of new collagen and elastin in the skin (when you heat the skin sufficiently, the collagen and elastin fibers shrink and tighten). How well they work, however, is a subject for debate. The amount of tightening varies greatly from patient to patient, and even in the best-case scenario, lasers won't correct *sagging* skin. "If you have skin laxity," says New York plastic surgeon Alan Matarasso, M.D., "you need to have it removed [surgically cut away] to see optimal results."

Thermage Thermage treatments, which can be performed on the face (to correct "turkey neck" and loose jowls), as well as the arms, tummy, thighs, and bum, use a radiofrequency laser to generate new collagen and tighten the skin in as little as one session. Results may appear gradually over a period of several months. Treatments may take anywhere from forty-five minutes to a little over an hour, and recovery time is minimal.

VelaShape VelaShape is an anticellulite treatment that uses a combination of radiofrequency laser, infrared light, and vacuum "massage" (basically, a special "roller" is massaged over the treatment area) to reduce the appearance of cellulite from the hips, thighs, stomach, and bum. (VelaShape treatments are not performed on the face.) The treatments are said to increase lymphatic drainage and reduce the size of fat cells; they also may help reduce the "circumference" of the thighs by an average of about an inch. Any results are temporary and must be maintained with repeat treatments.

THE PROCESS Thermage treatments are not generally painful, though treatments performed on the face may require local anesthesia. Slight swelling and redness is normal and may last for a few days. Bruising, however, is rare. VelaShape, on the other hand, requires no anesthesia; patients often describe the sensation as similar to that of a warm, deep massage. There is virtually no recovery time.

THE BILL Thermage treatments may range from $1,000 to $5,000, while VelaShape averages around $3,000 for a series of treatments.

What a Plastic Surgeon Can Do for You

THE BREASTS

Ah, the letdown (and I don't mean milk). During pregnancy, many of us—especially those of us with smaller chests—are at our most va-va-voom, since rising levels of estrogen and progesterone cause all the inner structures of the breast to grow. When we finally stop breastfeeding, however, two things happen: We lose fatty tissue, and the elastic fibers that support the breast off the chest wall have become stretched, resulting in an irreversible droop. Flat, pancake-like breasts can be a major bummer. Perhaps that's why more than three hundred thousand breast augmentations and more than one hundred thousand breast lifts were performed in 2009 alone.

There are two main problems that pregnancy may cause and which surgery can treat: sagging and loss of volume in the upper part of the breast (which occurs following the "deflation" of the breast post-pregnancy and/or breastfeeding). Sagging is generally alleviated via a mastopexy—or a breast lift, as it's more commonly known. The procedure is pretty much exactly what it sounds like: A surgeon lifts and repositions the breast higher up on the chest wall. Usually this involves cutting out excess skin and repositioning the nipple and areola.

"If the breast is lifted," explains Miami plastic surgeon Lee Gibstein, M.D., who specializes in breast work, "the nipple and areola have to be repositioned. That means you can't get away without a scar." Depending on the severity of your boob droop and the method your surgeon prefers, this could leave you with what's known as a "lollipop scar" (around the areola and down the center of the breast) or an "anchor scar" (around the areola, down the center, and under the breast crease). How well your body responds to scarring may be a factor in the procedure you opt to undergo. Speak to your doctor about the various methods he or she may use and what to expect once you've healed.

Some plastic surgeons contend that you can avoid scarring by getting an implant, a technically simpler operation where the scar is located under the breast crease and is usually barely noticeable. However, Dr. Gibstein (and other doctors who see lots of women postpartum) insists this doesn't work well. "If you augment [add an implant] but don't lift, the implant will sit in the right position, but the nipple will be too low on the breast mound,"

he says. Some women opt for what's called an augpexy, a combination lift and small augmentation. "Remember," says Dr. Gibstein, "implants add volume. Lifts make the breasts perkier. After breastfeeding, some women may need both."

It's not just the breasts that are affected post-baby. Many women may notice that their nipples are more elongated after breastfeeding and/or their areolae are larger and darker. Sometimes these changes are temporary. Sometimes they are not.

Nipple reduction It's a toe-curling thought, but it is possible to have the size of your nipples surgically reduced. "You can cut a bit off the top of the nipple, or you can cut a wedge from the middle, which may be a more elegant solution," says Dr. Gibstein. Nerve sensation is not usually lost, since the nerve that gives the nipple feeling is not in the nipple itself (the sensation comes from the lateral portion of the breast and courses up through the nipple, says Dr. Gibstein). However, it is possible for women who undergo a breast augmentation—even when the nipple is not repositioned—to lose sensation, since the nerve may be inadvertently damaged during the process of inserting and placing the actual implant. While most women who have nipple reductions can still breastfeed, there are no guarantees.

Areola reduction In an areola reduction, the surgeon will remove a circular rim of skin from within the pigmented areola—a thin circle within a circle—and then suture the breast back together. Many doctors recommend waiting at least a year after breastfeeding before considering any kind of nipple surgery, to see if the breast will return to its pre-pregnancy state on its own.

THE PROCESS Cosmetic breast surgery is a serious undertaking and requires quite a bit of planning. The surgery itself may take place in an outpatient or hospital setting; the majority of these procedures require general anesthesia. Many women go home the same day, though an overnight stay in a hospital is not uncommon.

For the first few days after surgery, you will experience swelling and bruising, and you will most likely feel *extremely* uncomfortable; your doctor will usually prescribe some kind of pain medication, which may make you a bit loopy. Without question, you will need child care

assistance for the first seventy-two hours (at an absolute minimum) following the procedure. The initial recovery may take one to two weeks, during which time you'll have limited mobility and won't be permitted to lift any heavy objects— including your children. Swelling will continue for several weeks, while general tenderness and soreness can linger for up to six months.

THE BILL Cosmetic breast surgery can run anywhere from $2,000 to $10,000, depending on the combination of treatments.

THE BELLY

Exercise is important. Core conditioning can make a monumental difference. But no amount of crunches or yoga poses will shrink loose, excess skin. So if your stomach resembles a shar-pei, it's not miraculously going to snap back. (The difference between excess fat and excess skin? Fat: You can grab it and knead it like bread. Skin can actually be pulled up and out; it rolls under your fingers.) New moms also may struggle with a stubborn little bulge in their lower abs, particularly if they had a C-section delivery. "The obstetrician is sewing you up, but your skin has not contracted yet, so you get this ledge—an overhang of skin over the scar," says Dr. Matarasso. The only complete fix for these kinds of problems is surgical. In other words, you're looking at an abdominoplasty.

Though there are several variations on the theme, an abdominoplasty, or tummy tuck, is basically the suturing together of the abdominal walls and the removal of excess skin to create a flat, pre-baby belly. In about 50 percent of cases, the procedure is combined with liposuction, the suctioning away of excess fat; lipo may also be performed on the back and flank to bring in the waist. Recent research from the University of Colorado, however, suggests a Whack-a-Mole complication: Liposuctioned fat may return within one year, though not to the spot where the procedure was performed. In the small study, women who had had liposuction on the lower abdomen, hips, or thighs saw a reaccumulation of fat in the upper abdomen and triceps.

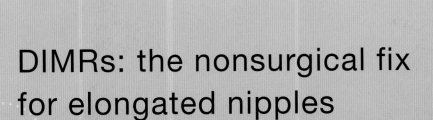

DIMRs: the nonsurgical fix for elongated nipples

If you're often embarrassed because your enlarged or elongated nipples sometimes show through clothing—and you can't bear the thought of or would never consider surgery—you may want to try DIMRS. (Yes, they're pronounced "dimmers," as in dimmers for the headlights. Get it?!) These reusable silicone pasties adhere to your bust without tape or adhesive (a few drops of water and your body heat activates the natural bond), so you'll never have to worry about flashing your high beams again. Around $30 at dimrs.com.

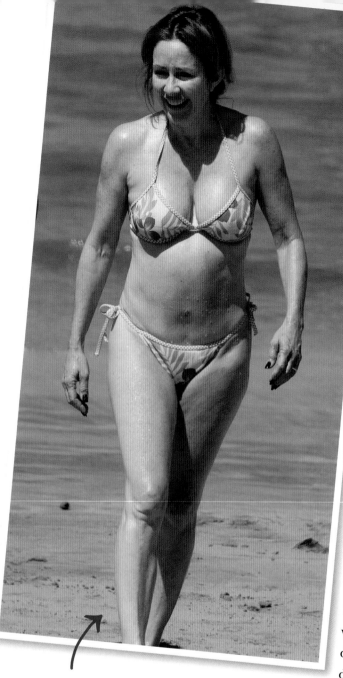

Actress Patricia Heaton admitted to having a tummy tuck and a breast lift after the birth of her fourth son.

THE PROCEDURE Much like cosmetic breast surgery, a tummy tuck is major surgery; it requires a significant amount of planning, and the recovery period can take weeks. Swelling, bruising, and pretty intense pain are all normal immediately following surgery. Your doctor will give you a prescription for pain medication, as well as detailed instructions on how to change and clean the dressings. You most likely will be asked to wear an abdominal support garment, too. Arrangements for child care are mandatory, as you'll be practically immobile for several weeks. Sitting as well as getting in and out of bed will be uncomfortable for a solid week, if not longer. Some women may choose to take as much as a month off work; strenuous exercise is not suggested for at least six weeks following surgery. And, of course, you'll have a permanent "smiley-face" scar from hip to hip, which, if you care about such things, will advertise to anyone who ever sees you down there that you had a big procedure done.

THE BILL The cost of a tummy tuck can range anywhere from $4,000 to $10,000 or even more.

the c-tuck: celebrity secret or urban myth?

For a few years now, rumors have been circulating the Internet that a growing number of celebrities are undergoing C-tucks immediately following childbirth—that is, a combination cesarean section and tummy tuck, to aid in the postpartum slim-down. Could this really be true?

Ladies, it's very likely that you can chalk this one up as a myth. There probably isn't a credible doctor alive who would admit to performing such a risky and unnecessary procedure as the C-tuck (at least not publicly). For one thing, the uterus is still swollen immediately following delivery (and will remain so for several weeks), so it would be nearly impossible to determine how much skin to remove. For another, adding an unnecessary surgery to a C-section may actually increase the risk of infection and postsurgical complications. In other words, it's just not safe. And last, a regular OB/GYN is simply not qualified to perform elective cosmetic surgery. Just because your abdomen has been opened up on the exam table doesn't make your delivery doctor somehow prepared to start hacking off excess fat and sagging skin. So if the C-tuck is more fiction than fact, what keeps all those baby blogs buzzing?

It seems the proliferation of the rumor can be attributed to three main points:

1. Celebrities seem to undergo elective C-sections at higher rates than the rest of us. That arouses suspicion. However, that notion is, of course, impossible to verify. Plenty of A-list actresses don't even feel comfortable divulging the details of their workout regimens or love lives, so it's perhaps silly to think they'd share the more intimate reasons for scheduling a C-section (ranging from the benign, like a breech baby, to the more severe, like preeclampsia) with the general public.

2. Celebrities are known to bounce back from childbirth faster than what we once thought possible. Hence, these women must be getting some kind of special voodoo in the delivery room, right? Unlikely. Celebrities do get preferential treatment, of course, in the form of personal nutrition counseling, personal training sessions, professional help from fashion experts, hair stylists, and makeup artists, even "celebrity wings" at hospitals—all services for which they pay a hefty fee. (As I've already pointed out, if we all had the resources that most celebrities do, we'd probably look pretty hot in a bathing suit, too.)

3. It is possible for a doctor to remove excess scar tissue incurred from previous C-sections while performing a current C-section. This procedure, however, should not be confused with an actual tummy tuck. Colloquially, it may sometimes be referred to as a "mini–tummy tuck," even though it's a vastly different procedure.

If an OB/GYN ever offers to give you a combination tummy tuck/C-section, the alarm bells should start ringing. Confirm just what it is he or she is suggesting, and if you're at all uncomfortable, consider switching to a different doctor.

THE VAGINA

Though "cosmetic-GYN"—or surgical procedures meant to beautify the vagina, of all things—is growing, it's a wildly controversial field and somewhat creepy arm of cosmetic surgery. As we discussed in chapter 1, many doctors feel these types of surgeries are unwarranted and unnecessary and that the doctors who perform them are preying on insecure women. A particularly terrifying article in *The Atlantic* even described a procedure referred to as "the Barbie," in which the labia minora are completely amputated to create a smooth genital appearance. Why on earth any woman would want to look like a plastic doll is beyond me. Nonetheless, because you might be curious (morbidly or otherwise) here's a rundown of the types of procedures available for your nether region. Proceed with caution.

Vaginoplasty The term *vaginoplasty* generally is used to describe any number of medical and cosmetic vaginal surgeries, of which there are tons; from the balloon vaginoplasty, for instance, which is a procedure that may be performed to correct an extremely rare congenital condition known as vaginal aplasia (essentially, the absence of a vagina), to something called penile inversion, which is a technique used in gender reassignment surgeries. For our purposes, however, vaginoplasty can be used to describe the nonreconstructive surgical tightening of the muscles that sometimes stretch and slacken with childbirth, resulting in a smaller, tighter vaginal canal—aka "vaginal rejuvenation." (This is not to be confused with the truly disturbing "revirginization" procedure, the surgical reconstruction of the hymen.) The surgery, which takes about an hour under general sedation, often may be combined with other pelvic repair procedures—for example, the repositioning of a prolapsed bladder. (Once there has been a weakening of the walls of the vagina, which partially support the bladder, the organ can fall partially into the vaginal canal. Depending on the severity of the condition, symptoms can range from a little urine leaking when you laugh to having a bladder that actually peeks out of the vagina—such a faux pas!)

Labiaplasty I know what you're probably thinking: Who's really concerned about the size and shape of her labia? Though I don't know a single woman who's ever discussed this issue with me, it seems lots of women care. Perhaps that's because the growing trend of "extreme bikini waxing" (from the landing strip to the full Brazilian) has rendered our private parts a lot less private. Add to that the ubiquity of the Internet—and, by extension, pornography—plus the frequency with which some young starlets "accidentally" get photographed without underwear, and it's easy to see why more and more women have discovered a new area of their body over which to obsess. Hooray.

Complicating matters are the unexpected, unplanned-for changes that can sometimes occur *down there*. I don't know that anyone's actually done a research study on labial changes after childbirth, but some women say their labia majora (the outer folds of skin) seem larger or "hang" more than before. Some dislike that their labia minora (inner folds) peek out from the majora, even though that's perfectly normal. And some feel insecure about the fact that their vagina is no longer perfectly symmetrical, even though that's perfectly normal, too. With the advent of so many surgically treated women out there (and lots of celebrity sex tapes floating around), we've somehow gotten the notion that it's "prettier" if "everything is sort of tucked in there neatly," as Dr. Gibstein describes it. Though I highly doubt that any of our mothers worried about having a "pretty" vagina.

For some women, there may be a bona fide medical reason to have the labia surgically reduced in size. "I had a patient with very large labia majora, and she was a bike racer," explains Dr. Gibstein. "After long hours of practice, the labia would be chafed and swollen, and sometimes they would bleed. It was incredibly uncomfortable, and having the skin cut away made it possible for her to race comfortably again." The majority of women, however, undergo the procedure for purely cosmetic reasons.

THE PROCESS Recovery for vaginoplasty and labiaplasty generally takes one to two weeks, during which time pain, swelling, and a small amount of bleeding are common. Women are advised to refrain from wearing a tampon and from sexual activity for at least six to eight weeks following surgery.

THE BILL The "Designer Vagina" will run you anywhere from $5,000 to $7,000. (Call me old-fashioned, I think that's money better spent on a 529 college fund.)

never, ever choose a plastic surgeon from the internet

Any doctor, of any repute, can pay a search engine to "optimize" his name so that it appears at the top of the list when you type in, say, "best plastic surgeon." Before and after pictures can be Photoshopped. One disgruntled (or insanely supportive) patient could write twenty "reviews" under different Internet handles. As if that weren't enough, competitive plastic surgeons have been known to anonymously trash *one another.* "It's the Wild West out there," confirms Dr. Matarasso. Here's what you need to know about choosing a qualified doctor.

Pay attention to credentials Unfortunately, any doctor can call him- or herself a "cosmetic surgeon." Your podiatrist could be a cosmetic surgeon; the term isn't regulated by any board or medical agency. (Same goes for titles like "beauty surgeon" or "aesthetic surgeon.") What you should be looking for is a "board-certified dermatologist" (for skin work including Botox injections, laser treatments, or chemical peels) or a "board-certified plastic surgeon" (for more invasive procedures, including tummy tucks and breast augmentations). In some cases, plastic surgeons spend more years in training than most other specialists, so the title and training really do matter. Your primary care physician should be able to give you a recommendation for a reputable surgeon in your area. Before scheduling a consultation with any physician, call the state medical board to confirm that his or her certifications are indeed up-to-date.

Next, it's time to find out how often your potential doctor has performed the procedure you're interested in having. If you want a tummy tuck, for example, you'll want a doctor who performs tummy tucks *at least* several times a month, not several times a year. So ask him. And while you're at it, ask to see before and after photos. Ask to see the surgical room. Ask anything and everything you can think of. If a doctor in any way makes light of your concerns, or doesn't answer a question to your satisfaction, drop everything and run.

Check out the surgical setting thoroughly These days, a large number of elective cosmetic procedures are performed in an outpatient setting (as opposed to a hospital room), from the minor, like Botox injections, to the more sophisticated, like breast implants and liposuction. And in large urban areas like New York City and Los Angeles—arguably the plastic surgery centers of America—some of the top doctors have sophisticated operating rooms in or near their offices; these are called "ambulatory surgical facilities," and they should be accredited either by state license or by a national body, such as the American Association for Accreditation of Ambulatory Surgery Facilities. While it's rare that an elective procedure would be performed in an inpatient setting, some patients with systemic diseases or medical conditions require hospitalization and additional monitoring.

Speak to your doctor about which surgical setting is best suited for your procedure. If an outpatient facility is recommended, make sure that it's accredited and ask if your doctor has hospital privileges at a nearby medical institution, so that he or she may admit you if the need arises.

Confessions of a Hollywood Mom

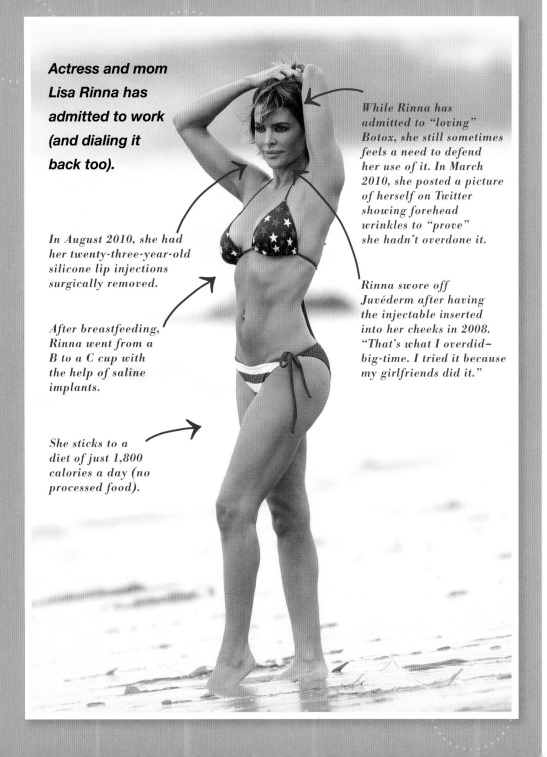

Actress and mom Lisa Rinna has admitted to work (and dialing it back too).

In August 2010, she had her twenty-three-year-old silicone lip injections surgically removed.

After breastfeeding, Rinna went from a B to a C cup with the help of saline implants.

She sticks to a diet of just 1,800 calories a day (no processed food).

While Rinna has admitted to "loving" Botox, she still sometimes feels a need to defend her use of it. In March 2010, she posted a picture of herself on Twitter showing forehead wrinkles to "prove" she hadn't overdone it.

Rinna swore off Juvéderm after having the injectable inserted into her cheeks in 2008. "That's what I overdid— big-time. I tried it because my girlfriends did it."

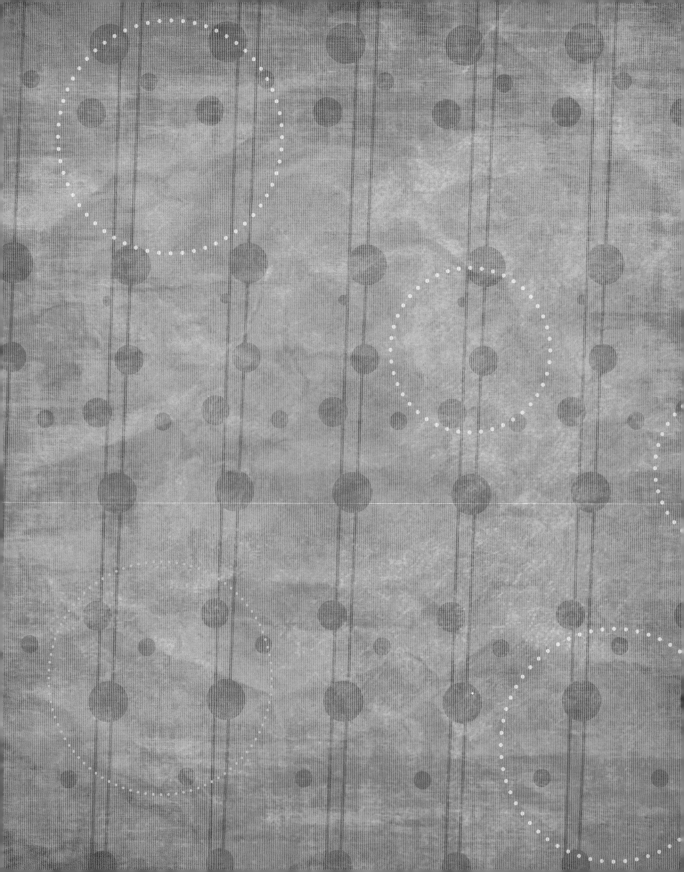

afterword

Isn't it funny, after everything we put ourselves through to "bounce back" after giving birth, that so many of us are eager to go back and do it again?

I was filled with fear—actual terror—before giving birth to my first son, Will, consumed with worry over the physical agony I was sure childbirth would involve. I couldn't wrap my head around the idea that, somehow, eight pounds or so of wriggly, writhing newborn was going to get itself out of a teeny-tiny hole. As someone whose whole career centers on creating deadlines, meeting deadlines, and sometimes moving deadlines, I also completely freaked out that this was one appointment I would not be able to change; it was happening whether I was ready or not. But then sometime around the eighth month of pregnancy, I had had it—I needed this baby out of me. I was ridiculously uncomfortable and, by that point, improbably huge. A random person on the street asked if I was expecting twins; others assumed I was overdue. I must have looked as miserable as I felt. In fact, one colleague told me that he had observed me walking down the hallway from behind—and that I looked like a steamship slowly drifting down a river. This is not a flattering analogy.

Then, the time came. It was a Monday, and Jennifer Lopez had just gotten married. I stayed at work until two A.M. to finish the cover story about her wedding; five hours later, I was on the *Today* show talking about it. Immediately afterward (and completely exhausted), I dragged myself to my doctor's office for my weekly visit. After having been misdiagnosed the week before, they discovered that, yes, my water was leaking. I had to go straight to the hospital to be induced. Suddenly, I had to confront every last fear I'd been concocting over the previous nine months. My face must have gone totally white when the doctor told me she'd be right back with the "amnio hook." (On the flip side, that epidural needle in the back didn't seem so bad compared to the pain it was going to take away.) When it was finally time to push, I thought my head might explode. I actually wondered if my eyes could pop out of my skull from the strain of pushing. Childbirth is one

instance where what you see on TV is no embellishment; women really do scream like wild animals. I also could not get one of the most horrifying parts of *What to Expect When You're Expecting* out of my mind: that some women actually poop on the table. (Luckily, I did not.) To top everything off, I was at New York University Medical Center, a teaching hospital; different residents kept popping in to watch, and I was terror-stricken that someone I knew from college—perhaps some guy I hadn't seen in years—would appear at my feet and see all my private parts.

Finally, after ninety minutes of agonizing pushing and near delirium, my son finally popped out, and it was the most incredible feeling of sheer joy…and physical relief. While I nervously watched the doctors perform routine tests under heat lamps, I begged my husband to get me a Coke—having had gestational diabetes, it was my first taste of sugar in months. (TMI, I promptly threw it up.) Even after all that, and even though I wouldn't have dared utter the words to my husband, I knew, right then and there, that I wanted to do it all again. And I kept that thought close throughout the whirlwind twenty-four hours that followed—even when my son bit down so hard on my nipple that a nurse had to teach me how to get him to release his pit bull death vise; even when I had to clean up the natural disaster–like oil spill of meconium in the middle of the night. It was a high I had never known in my life. There was once a very funny headline on the website for the satirical newspaper the *Onion*, something like MAN DESCRIBES MIRACLE OF 8 BILLIONTH BIRTH ON EARTH. Because, yes, tens of thousands of women give birth every day, everywhere. But when it happens to you, the elation is indescribable.

I've always joked that the *real* miracle, though, is that anyone ever produces a second baby after having the first one. After all, there is often so much tension and anxiety between the parents for those first few months; everyone in the family is so wiped out. And let's be honest, there's usually not a lot of romance going on that first year. Add to that the general sort of weirdness that comes with raising a baby. There were times when my husband, who is truly one of the kindest, sweetest people I've ever known, could not bear to be in the same room with me while I was pumping; that awful wheezing sound of the machine completely grossed him out. Lots of really unsexy stuff goes on once you've become a mother. Still, plenty of us, after finally getting our bodies (and our homes) back into something resembling a presentable

state, choose to do it all again. And again. And, sometimes, *again.*

It was perhaps fitting that—right around the time I was putting the finishing touches on this book—I learned that I was pregnant with my third child, this time a little girl. As I type these words, I feel enormously excited and, of course, cripplingly exhausted. And even though I know that I am about to re-enter that black hole of dirty diapers, sleepless nights, compulsive visits to the bathroom scale, and idiotic guilt over not making my own baby food, I also feel tremendous gratitude. I'm older now, so I'm thrilled that I will get to experience childbirth one more time, and—finally!—I now know what to expect while I'm expecting.

Without a doubt, having children has made me a better person. I am far less judgmental and mentally forgive people for shortcomings all the time. (Why's that guy such a jerk? Because he had a terrible childhood!) At home, I'm very conscious not to call someone or something ugly or stupid or anything else insulting in my kids' presence (and hopefully not even when they aren't around). I *try* not to raise my voice (emphasis on "try") and to take the time to explain every last thing about which they are curious.

And they are definitely curious. My

eldest son—a second-grader as I write this—calls it like he sees it. One recent morning he woke up and crawled into bed with us. He was looking at my face and said, "Why is grown-up skin so wrinkly and spotty?" Mere days later, he was looking at my legs in shorts while we were reading a book on his bed and he asked, "Why do you have such big legs?" I realize that he's not saying this to be insulting or mean, since he is neither; they're just his casual observations. Of course, he and his little brother, Tate, manage to come up with some rather practical questions too: Why do you wear lipstick? Why do you curl your lashes with that thing? Why do you wear high heels when you know they hurt your feet? Why do girls paint their toenails?

When these questions are asked through the eyes of a child, you begin to see the absurdity in what we as women do. (Why would I use some strange forcepslike instrument to, of all things, *curl my eyelashes*?!) Sometimes I even feel resentful about all these strange, time-sucking rituals that women accept as both necessary and normal…yet I do them anyway. It's to those types of questions that I usually stumble around for an answer. The wrong answer would be something like "Because your mother looks like crap in the morning." Usually I'll say something like "It's just the way women get ready" or, if I'm especially tired, "Mommies are silly." I don't know if that's the right answer. All I know is that I feel better when I look better.

In the summer of 2010, my family and I moved to Los Angeles and I became editor of a publication called the *Hollywood Reporter*. We cover the entertainment industry rather than the lives (and looks) of celebrities, so it's more who-directed-what-movie than who's-dating-who. The change has been a bit of a mental relief. Sometimes I just don't need to know how someone lost the baby weight. Or who wore it better. Or how to get a bikini body in a week and a half. The level of celebrity obsession on those sorts of details is fun—yes—but it can be exhausting.

I admit, I was a little nervous when I began work on *How to Look Hot in a Minivan;* I didn't want it to be thought of as superficial or frivolous or antifeminist or silly. I didn't want women to feel I was leading the charge to the plastic surgeon's office or suggesting that a postnatal stomach sag was something to be ashamed of. Personally, I think the trend of "mommy makeovers" and unbridled celebrity worship takes its toll on our collective self-esteem. And after the move from the "intellectual capital" of the country (New York City) to the center of celebrity (Los Angeles), I sometimes worry that my children will be affected, too. (I was shocked when one of them started pressing me on the box office performance of *Puss in Boots*, the other day; they absorb *everything*.) And I most definitely don't want them to be looks-obsessed. I know I will be nothing short of crestfallen the first time they make fun of a woman's looks, or comment on her breasts, or call someone fat, or make fun of someone's clothes, but I know it will happen. Despite my best efforts.

In Tina Fey's book *Bossypants*, she included a chapter called "All Girls Must Be Everything" in which she enumerates the laundry list of attributes that a woman must have to qualify as beautiful these days: "Now, if you're not 'hot,' you are expected to work on it until you are ... If you don't have a good body, you'd better starve the body you have down to a neutral shape, then bolt on some breast implants, replace your teeth, dye your skin orange, inject your lips, sew on some hair and call yourself the Playmate of the Year." Rhetorically, she jokes: "How do we survive this? How do we teach our daughters and our gay sons that they are good enough the way they are? We have to lead by example."

Of course, that's often easier said than done. We've all felt the pressures to look as good as possible, to be as thin as possible.

(In fact, a recent survey of new moms revealed that 25 percent felt like they were competing with other mothers—and with celebrities—to see who could drop their baby weight first.) And we live in a very, very strange world, a world where a sex tape can net you (and your entire family, apparently) a reality TV empire, where women regularly cart pictures of famous people's sloped noses and perfect pouts to the surgeon's office and demand to be made over in the image of someone else, where a misguided mother may or may not have been performing Botox injections on her plucky eight-year-old daughter before blabbing about it to an audience of millions on *Good Morning America*, where the *New York Times* devoted an entire story not just to the hot mom phenomenon, but to the hot *grandma* phenomenon. ("Glam-mas," they called them.) One of the more appalling stories we covered at the *Hollywood Reporter* was about a short-lived reality show called *Bridalplasty*. You may remember this—it was about women competing for full-body plastic surgery makeovers before their impending weddings. The message? You have to "fix" yourself before you even walk down the aisle!

I don't know what this really means for us or for our children. It certainly can't be healthy. But to me, there is a difference between losing all perspective and just wanting to feel good about the way you look. I try not to freak out too much about these things, but (like everyone else) I have my moments. Shortly after turning forty, I made an appointment with a personal trainer at my local gym. In the course of the first session, he looked at me and asked: "How old are you? About forty?" It was like a kick in the gut—I don't think anyone had ever correctly guessed my age my entire life. I was reeling. *Oh, my God, what makes me look forty? How can I fix this?* I came home, still traumatized, and told my husband that my trainer thought I was forty. To which he said, "But you *are* forty." Reality check. (Thanks, husband!)

So, yes, we live in a nutty world where women are supposed to constantly engineer themselves to look younger, better, and sexier. It's insanity. At the same time, it doesn't seem particularly helpful to pretend that childbirth and motherhood doesn't turn your world—and your body—upside down. The pressure to pretend that it's all so easy might be just as unhealthy as the pressure women sometimes feel to look like Heidi Klum. I wanted to write a book that, first and foremost, took an honest look at this crazy societal shift we all have been subjected to, one where the fundamental perception of what a mother should look

like has been completely transformed. And I hope that by giving women access to the various experts I've met over the course of my career, I've helped explain a simple fact: All new mothers—even the most famous— need some help bouncing back after baby. It's normal to feel pudgy and plump and exhausted and unattractive in the weeks and months following delivery. But the pros who work with those headline-making celebrity moms can simplify, demystify, and share some seriously helpful secrets for looking (and feeling) better. That kind of information is not the birthright of the rich and famous.

In more ways than I care to admit, I *am* the crazy mother that I mention time and again throughout this book, the one who obsesses over her kids, compares herself in vain with celebrities, and martyrs herself to make sure everyone in the family is taken care of before she is. But it's on those crazy, stressful days that I remind myself: No one has ever come up short by being a little more informed, by dabbling in self-improvement, and by practicing moderation. Sometimes a stolen afternoon at the spa or an indulgent haircut in an expensive salon or even just an hour alone to sweat it out on the treadmill is enough to remind us that taking pride in the way we look can send a *positive* message to our children. Moms are important, too.

acknowledgments

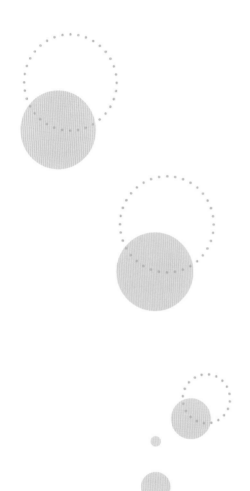

I'd always loved the idea of writing a book, but didn't have the faintest idea how to get one done.

Back in 2007, when I was still working as the editor of *Us Weekly,* a book agent by the name of David Kuhn asked me to lunch after he read a profile of me in the *New York Observer.* The story touched on the explosion of "babymania" due to the American obsession with celebrity culture. (Indeed, 2007 went down on record as the year most babies were born in the United States. Ever.) In the piece the writer Tom Wolfe was quoted as saying, "The motif of babies and the bump is just rampant. Brad and Angelina and Britney and Kevin [Federline], it's all about babies. The one thing that *Us Weekly* has done that's a great boost to the nation is, they've probably increased the birthrate."

Two years later, I called David with the idea for this book. He "got it" right away, and I am grateful for his enthusiasm and guidance in conceiving it.

Creating a book is about making your own life an open book, and my editor, Kathryn Huck at St. Martin's Press, pushed me gently yet firmly to be personal and revealing in ways my more guarded nature might not otherwise have allowed. John Murphy, director of publicity at St. Martin's, was also a confidence builder: I relaxed during this process when, over breakfast one morning, he told me that an early draft (that he'd read without my knowledge) was not just fun but also funny, and that he loved it. I could tell he believed in it—which made me believe in it, too.

Between my day job and parenting duties, completing this book was not easy. The creation of any book is a lonely, anxiety-filled process, and I was blessed to have found Courtney Hargrave, who had the talent, perseverance, and patience to take my interviews and random thoughts and organize them into cohesive, clever language. She was a tremendous ally and sounding board throughout the entire process. Simply said, this book would not exist without her.

Also, I could not have done this without the aid of various people: Jann Wenner for giving me the freedom and opportunity to make *Us Weekly*, in its heyday, into what I wanted; to my busy longtime friends (and fellow mothers) Nuna Alberts, Caroline Schaefer, and Jennifer Savarese for actually reading the entire book early and giving advice; to *Hollywood Reporter* design director

Shanti Marlar and photo director Jennifer Laski for lending their time and critical eye; to *Us Weekly* photo director Jennifer Halper and *Hollywood Reporter* senior photo producer Carrie Smith for helping me all the time, any time; and to Lisa Dallos for her wisdom and enthusiasm.

There are reporters and journalists I've known throughout my career whose knowledge and experience informed this book. Jennifer O'Neill, Jessica Mehalic, Judith Newman, Marisa Fox, and *Hollywood Reporter* fashion editor Carol McColgin all contributed their expertise; in addition, *Us Weekly* fashion director Sasha Charnin Morrison and beauty director Gwen Flamberg pointed me toward many of the experts quoted in the book; earlier in my life, they'd also helped me to not look like a total mess during my postnatal haze and I am forever indebted.

Last but not least, I say thank you to my own mother, who instilled self-esteem without ever pushing me to be obsessed with my appearance, and certainly never had a nanny, time to go to the gym, or money that she wouldn't rather spend on her children than herself. And I am forever, constantly grateful for my husband, without whose devotion I would not have found the time to sit down at a computer, and whose skills, patience, and kindness as a parent know no bounds.

photo credits

All Photography by Michael Pirrocco, except:

x: (top left) Paul Hiffmeyer/Disney Parks via Getty Images; (top center) Stefanie Keenan/Getty Images; (top right) Kevin Mazur/Getty Images; (center left) Jason Merritt/Getty Images; (center) DS-ISM/LA-Tom/Flynet; (bottom left) TRB/Fame Pictures; (bottom center) Sara Jaye Weiss; (bottom right) Jake Holly/startraksphoto.com. 3: Sara Jaye Weiss. 4: Kevin Mazur/Getty Images. 8: (left) ©BAUER-GRIFFIN.COM; (right) Jason LaVeris/FilmMagic. 9: (clockwise from far left): Evan Agostini/BEImages; Jordan Strauss/WireImage; Steve Granitz/WireImage; Michael Stewart/Film Magic; Dimitrios Kambouris/WireImage; Barry Talesnick/Retna. 10: Getty Images. 12: Frazer Harrison/Getty Images. 16: Stephen Lovekin/Getty Images. 19: INFphoto.com. 22: Stefanie Keenan/Getty Images. 25: ©BAUER-GRIFFIN.COM. 26: Paul Viant/Getty Images. 30: (left) Jason Mitchell/BuzzFoto/FilmMagic; (center) Homero Tercero/WENN; (top right) Newscom; (bottom right) Zach Bloom/BuzzFoto/FilmMagic. 31: (top left) Mario Magnani/Getty Images; (top center) Donna Ward/Getty Images; (top right) Dimitrios Kambouris/WireImage; (bottom left) Sam Sharma/Nathanael Jones/PacificCoastNews/Newscom; (bottom center) Mel Bouzad/FilmMagic; (bottom right) Tim Graham/Getty Images. 32: (left) Chris Jackson–Pool/Getty Images; (top right) Fame pictures; (bottom right) JCalderon/Splash News/Newscom. 33: (left) Jesse Grant/WireImage; (top right) MAC/Fame Pictures; (bottom right) John M. Heller/Getty Images. 34: (top left) Leon Neal/AFP/Getty Images; (bottom left) Christy Bowe/Polaris; (right) REUTERS/Jonathan Ernst. 35: (top left) LUIS ACOSTA/AFP/Getty Images; (top right) Gary Fabiano/Pool via Bloomberg/Getty Images; (bottom left) Win McNamee/Getty Images; (bottom right) Olivier Douliery/Abaca Press/MCT/Newscom. 36:

(top) XPOSUREPHOTOS.COM; (bottom left) James Devaney/WireImage; (right) Kristina Sazonova/Epsilon/Getty Images. 37: (left) Headlinephoto/BuzzFoto/FilmMagic; (center) Todd Williamson/Getty Images; (right) PER/Fame Pictures. 39: (right) John Shearer/WireImage. 40: (right) Splash News. 41: (right) Deano/SDFL/Splash News. 42: (right) Jackson Lee/Splash News. 43: (right) Gotcha Images/Splash News. 44: (right) Gustavo Caballero/Getty Images. 45: (right) Kevin Parry/WireImage. 46: (right) Castro/PacificCoastNews/Newscom. 47: (right) Doug Meszler/Splash News. 48: (right) Nancy Rivera/ACEPIXS.COM. 54: Ray Tamarra/Getty Images. 58: Fame Pictures. 60: Frazer Harrison/Getty Images. 61: (top) Stefanie Keenan/Getty Images; (center) Francois Durand/Getty Images. 62: (bottom) courtesy of Spanx. 64: courtesy of Spanx. 67: Brian Prahl/Splash News. 70: Robert Houser/Getty Images. 74: (top) Sara De Boer/Retna Ltd.; (center) Michael Kovac/FilmMagic; (bottom) Mike Coppola/FilmMagic. 75: Mike Coppola/FilmMagic. 76: Kevin Winter/Getty Images. 77: (left) Tony Barson/WireImage; (right) Michael N. Todaro/FilmMagic. 78: (top left) Olivier Douliery/ABACAUSA.COM/Newscom; (top right) Nicholas Kamm/AFP/Getty Images; (bottom left) Richard Corkery/NY Daily News Archive/Getty Images; (bottom right) Bennett Raglin/Getty Images. 79: Dimitrios Kambouris/WireImage. 80: courtesy of Oscar Blandi. 81: (top) iStock; (bottom) Steve Granitz/WireImage. 82: (top) Jeffrey Mayer/WireImage; (bottom) courtesy of TouchBack. 83: Ian Gavan/Getty Images. 84: (top) Jackson Lee/Splash News/Newscom; (center) Frazer Harrison/Getty Images; (bottom) Jean Baptiste Lacroix/WireImage. 87: (left) Steve Granitz/WireImage; (right) Randy Brooke/FilmMagic. 88: (top) Big Stock; (bottom) courtesy of L'Oreal. 89: (left) courtesy of Clairol; (top right) Big Stock; (bottom right) courtesy of John Frieda. 90: courtesy of Garnier. 93: Ethan Miller/Getty Images. 94: Lester Cohen/WireImage. 96: Jeffrey Mayer/WireImage. 97: (left) courtesy of T3; (right) courtesy of Pantene. 98-101: Photos by Gabrielle Revere. 102: Jamie Grill/Getty Images. 105: Jordan Strauss/WireImage. 107: iStock. 108: (top) Michael N. Todaro/FilmMagic; (bottom) Jason Merritt/Getty Images. 109: (top) Robin Platzer/Twin Images; (bottom) Steve Granitz/Getty Images. 110: Tooga Productions, Inc./Getty Images. 111: (top) Junko Kimura/Getty Images; (bottom)

Jordan Strauss/Getty Images. 112: (top) Chance Yeh/PatrickMcMullan.com/Sipa Press/Newscom; (bottom) Jordan Strauss/WireImage. 113: iStock. 116: Jordan Strauss/FilmMagic. 117: Kevin Mazur/WireImage. 118: Joy Scheller/iPhoto. 119: courtesy of La Roche-Posay. 120: courtesy of Dr. Hauschka. 121: (top) courtesy of Laura Mercier; (bottom) courtesy of Yves Saint Laurent. 122: (left) courtesy of Josie Maran; (right) courtesy of Era Rayz. 124: courtesy of Blinc. 125: (left) courtesy of Smith's; (right) courtesy of Lipstick Queen. 126: (left) courtesy of Shiseido; (right) courtesy of Benefit. 128: courtesy of Essence of Beauty. 129: Steve Wisbauer/Getty Images. 130: Venturelli/Getty Images. 131: Stephen Lovekin/Getty Images. 132: Alexandra Grablewski/Getty Images. 135: PAUL J. RICHARDS/AFP/Getty Images. 137: Getty Images. 138: (left) Larry Hill/ZUMA Press/Newscom; (right) Eaglepress. 139: (top left) Junko Kimura/Getty Images; (top right) Tony Barson/WireImage; (bottom left) Jim Spellman/WireImage; (bottom right) VIPIX/©2007 Ramey Photo. 141: Geraldina Amaya/Frank Ross Media. 143: (left) iStock; (right) iStock. 145: (center left) Big Stock; (all others) iStock. 149: Davies and Starr. 152: iStock. 153: Brian Hagiwara/Getty Images. 156: iStock. 157: iStock. 158: Erika McConnell Photography. 160: (left) Embassy Pictures/Courtesy Neal Peters Collection; (right) Universal Pictures/Courtesy Neal Peters Collection. 161: Chris Haston/NBC via Getty Images. 162: (left) ©www.splashnews.com; (right) Dimitrios Kambouris/WireImage. 163: (top) GSI Media; (bottom left) ©www.splashnews.com; (bottom center) Flynetpictures.com; (bottom right) Jeff Kravitz/FilmMagic. 164: Matthew Symons/Coleman-Ryder. 168-171: Photos by Cory Sorensen. 172: Kevin Mazur/Getty Images. 174: iStock. 175: iStock. 179: Steve Wisbauer/Getty Images. 180: (left) Jeff Kravitz/FilmMagic; (right) Andrew H. Walker/Getty Images. 181: Soul Brother/FilmMagic. 186: Paul Bradbury/Getty Images. 190: Jason Merritt/Getty Images. 191: Michael Loccisano/Getty Images. 192: iStock. 193: iStock. 197: iStock. 200: Starsurf/Splash News. 205: Albert Michael/startraksphoto.com.

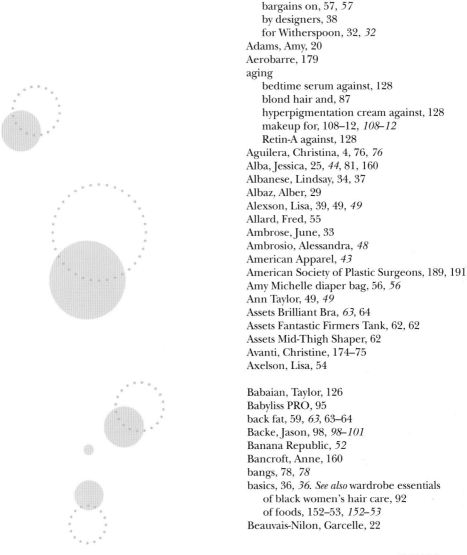

index